Measurement of Nursing Outcomes

Second Edition

Volume 2:
Client Outcomes and Quality of Care

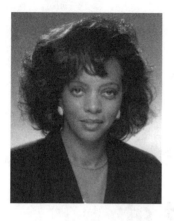

Ora L. Strickland, PhD, RN, FAAN, is a Research Scientist at the Atlanta Veterans Administration Medical Center and is Professor in the Nell Hodgson Woodruff School of Nursing at Emory University in Atlanta, Georgia. She earned a doctoral degree in child development and family relations from the University of North Carolina, Greensboro; a master's degree in maternal and child health nursing from Boston University, Massachusetts; and, received a bachelor's degree in nursing from North Carolina Agricultural and Technical State University, Greensboro.

Dr. Strickland co-edited the original four volumes of *Measurement of Nursing Outcomes*. She is the founder and senior editor of the *Journal of Nursing Measurement*. An internationally known specialist in nursing research, measurement, evaluation, maternal and child health and parenting, Dr. Strickland has published widely in professional journals and is frequently called upon as a consultant by health care agencies, universities, government agencies, and community organizations. She has presented more than 200 public lectures, speeches and workshops, and her research has been featured in newspapers, magazines, and on radio and television.

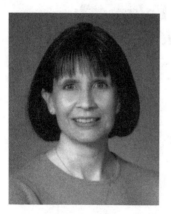

Colleen DiIorio, PhD, RN, FAAN, is a Professor in the Department of Behavioral Sciences and Health Education at Rollins School of Public Health, Emory University and Department of Family and Community Nursing in the Nell Hodgson Woodruff School of Nursing, at Emory University. Dr. DiIorio earned a doctoral degree in nursing research and theory development from New York University. She received her master's degree in nursing, with a functional minor in delivery of nursing services, from New York University and received a bachelor's degree in nursing from the University of Iowa.

Dr. DiIorio has extensive experience in health promotion research. She currently serves as principal investigator on four NIH funded research grants. Her work covers two broad areas addressing health behavior and behavioral change: adherence/self-management and HIV prevention. Dr. DiIorio has published numerous articles and chapters on self-management and HIV prevention in addition to topics on measurement, health promotion, disease prevention, and evaluation. Dr. DiIorio has served as a consultant to and on panels of community organizations, governmental agencies, and professional organizations. She currently serves as associate editor of the *Journal of Nursing Measurement*.

Measurement of Nursing Outcomes

Second Edition

Volume 2:
Client Outcomes and Quality of Care

Ora Lea Strickland, PhD, RN, FAAN
Colleen Dilorio, PhD, RN, FAAN
Editors

 Springer Publishing Company

Springer Publishing Company, Inc.
536 Broadway
New York, NY 10012-3955

Acquisitions Editor: Ruth Chasek
Production Editor: Pamela Lankas
Cover design by Joanne Honigman

03 04 05 06 07 / 5 4 3 2 1

Library of Congress Cataloging-in-Publication Data

Measurement of nursing outcomes / Ora L. Strickland, Colleen DiIorio, editors,—2nd ed.
    p. cm.
    Includes bibliographical references and index.
    ISBN 0-8261-1427-X (v. 2)
        1. Nursing—Standards. 2. Nursing audit. I. Strickland, Ora L.
    II. DiIorio, Colleen.
        [DNLM: 1. Nursing—methods. 2. Clinical Competence.
    3. Nursing—standards. 4. Outcome and Process Assessment (Health Care). WY 16 M484 2001]
    RT85.5 .M434 2001
    610.73—so21
                                  00-054928

Printed in the United States of America by Sheridan Books Inc.

Contents

Preface

This volume of the *Measurement of Nursing Outcomes* book series provides nursing measurement tools that focus on client outcomes and quality of care. It updates and expands upon the original four volumes produced in 1988 and 1990 that were co-edited by Carolyn F. Waltz and Ora L. Strickland. The major purposes of this publication are to:

1. Keep client-focused nursing instruments easily accessible to those who need to use them;
2. Update some of the instruments that appeared in the original volumes by providing additional psychometric information; and
3. Encourage the dissemination of other nursing measures that are useful to the practice of nurse clinicians and researchers.

Over the past twenty years, much progress has been made in nursing measurement. The first four volumes of the *Measurement of Nursing Outcomes* book series were a direct outgrowth of the Measurement of Clinical and Educational Nursing Outcomes Project, which was funded by the Division of Nursing, Special Projects Branch, Department of Health and Human Services Grant 1D10NU23085. Over 200 nurse educators and researchers sharpened their skills in nursing measurement through this project by developing or modifying and testing tools to measure nursing outcome variables. The skills that these nurses garnered through this project have not only increased the number of quality nursing measures, but have improved the quality of measurement content taught in nursing programs. Given the recent focus on evidenced-based outcomes, progress made in this area has had a significant impact on nursing practice, quality of care assessment, and knowledge development and scholarship in the field.

This publication serves as a distinct representation of the progress made in the advancement of nursing measurement during the past decade and ushers the field into the twenty-first century with more stellar measurement instruments that better quantify key concepts and constructs that are important to nursing practice and research. It is presented with the full recognition that nurses can provide the best of care, conduct the most potent and influential research, and effectively expand the profession's knowledge base when their approaches to quantifying nursing variables are dependable, that is, measure the phenomena of interest reliably and accurately. In essence, consistent and appropriate application of measurement principles and practices, along with the development of sensitive and valid measures, is crucial if the profession of nursing is to continue to advance and impact patient care.

A variety of instruments that address concepts relevant to client outcomes and quality of care are presented in this volume. Several of the measures are disease specific and have been designed for use in diseases such as heart disease, cancer, or multiple sclerosis. Several of the instruments have been designed specifically for assessing function and activities in older persons. This is quite timely given that the segment of the population in the United States that is growing most rapidly is that of older Americans. Several of the tools can be used with clients in the general population or with various health care conditions. In general, the instruments included in this volume address three topical areas: Measuring Functional Abilities and Outcomes of Care, Client's Perceptions of Care, and Measuring Care and Quality of Care. It is our hope that the dissemination of these measurement tools will not only facilitate better outcome assessment and knowledge development, but will encourage their use and their further development and testing, thereby advancing the state of nursing measurement even further. Although we have come a long way in nursing measurement, work in the area needs to continue. The strides forward that we have made thus far do not negate the fact that we still have far to go and much work to be done.

ORA LEA STRICKLAND, PhD, RN, FAAN
COLLEEN DiIORIO, PhD, RN, FAAN

Acknowledgment

The editors gratefully acknowledge Regina M. Daniel, Administrative Assistant in the Rollins School of Public Health at Emory University, who graciously contributed her time and management skills to ensure the completion of this book. Her commitment, perseverance, and talents were liberally shared during the development of this book. Thank you, Regina. You are greatly appreciated.

Acknowledgment

[faded, illegible text]

Contributors

Marion E. Broome, PhD, RN, FAAN
Professor and Associate Dean for Research
School of Nursing
University of Alabama at Birmingham
Birmingham, Alabama

Kathleen C. Buckwalter, PhD, RN, FAAN
Associate Provost for Health Sciences
Professor, College of Nursing
The University of Iowa
Iowa City, Iowa

Shirley Metz Caldwell, EdD, RNC
Retired
Sumas, Washington

Jennifer Cutler, BScN, RN
Research Associate
Faculty of Nursing
University of Toronto
Toronto, Ontario, Canada

Pam Dawson
Past (Retired) Director,
Collaborative Research Program
Long Term Care
Toronto, Ontario, Canada

Lillian Eriksen, DSN, RN
University of Texas-Houston
Health Sciences Center
School of Nursing
Houston, Texas

Janet I. Feldman, PhD, RN
Vice President, Qualitas Associates
Downers Grove, Illinois

Jeanne Flannery, DSN, ARNP, CNRN, CRRN, CCH
Professor, School of Nursing
The Florida State University
Tallahassee, Florida

Elsie E. Gulick, PhD, RN, FAAN
Professor, College of Nursing
Rutgers, The State University of New Jersey
Newark, New Jersey

Alicia Huckstadt, PhD, APRN, BC, FNP
Professor and Graduate Program Director
The Wichita State University
Wichita, Kansas

Debra A. Jansen, PhD, RN
Associate Professor
University of Wisconsin-Eau Claire
School of Nursing
Eau Claire, Wisconsin

Mary L. Keller, PhD, RN
Associate Professor
University of Wisconsin-Madison
School of Nursing
Madison, Wisconsin

Imogene M. King, EdD, RN, FAAN
Retired
South Pasadena, Florida

Gene W. Marsh, PhD, RN
Associate Professor
University of Colorado Health
    Sciences Center
Denver, Colorado

Anna M. McDaniel, DNS, RN
Associate Professor
Department of Environments for
    Health
Indiana University
School of Nursing
Indianapolis, Indiana

Ptlene Minick, PhD, RN
Georgia State University
School of Nursing
Atlanta, Georgia

Teri Mobley, BSN, RN
Project Coordinator, Center for
    Nursing Research
School of Nursing
University of Alabama at
    Birmingham
Birmingham, Alabama

Woodrow W. Morris, PhD
Emeritus Professor and Former
    Associate Dean
College of Medicine
The University of Iowa
Iowa City, Iowa

Robert J. Richard, MA
Kentfield, California

Karen R. Robinson, PhD, RN, FAAN
Associate Director for Clinical
    Operations
Department of Veterans Affairs
    Medical Center
Fargo, North Dakota

Anna L. Schwartz, PhD, ARNP
Associate Professor
Oregon Health Sciences
    University
Portland, Oregon

Souraya Sidani, PhD, RN
Associate Professor
Faculty of Nursing
University of Toronto
Toronto, Ontario, Canada

Jean C. Toth, DNSc, RN, CNS,
    BCC
Associate Professor of
    Cardiovascular Nursing
The Catholic University of
    America
Washington, DC

Gwen van Servellen, PhD, RN
Professor and Chair, Acute Care
    Section
School of Nursing
University of California, Los
    Angeles
Los Angeles, California

Donna L. Wells, PhD, RN
Associate Professor & Associate
    Dean, Education
Chair, Graduate Department of
    Nursing Science
Faculty of Nursing
University of Toronto
Toronto, Ontario, Canada

Nancy Wells, DNS, RN
Director of Nursing Research
Research Associate Professor
Vanderbilt University Medical
    Center
Nashville, Tennessee

Kathleen Wheeler, PhD, APRN
Associate Professor and Director
    of the Graduate Program
Fairfield University
Fairfield, Connecticut

Judi Witter
Director, Performance Assessment
    and Improvement
Carondelet St. Mary's Hospital
Tucson, Arizona

PART I
Measuring Functional Abilities and Outcomes of Care

1

Assessment of Functional Abilities and Goal Attainment Scales: A Criterion-Referenced Measure

Imogene M. King

This chapter discusses the Criterion-Referenced Measure of Goal Attainment Tool, a measure of functional abilities and goal attainment.

PURPOSE

Standards of nursing practice are generated for the purpose of providing professional nursing care for patients and measuring outcomes of nursing care. Among these outcomes are those that indicate attainment of a state of health consistent with an individual's and a family's ability to function in their usual roles, such as teacher, administrator, mother, and father. Determining whether or not a standard is met is contingent on evaluating the outcome(s) associated with that standard. The criteria used for outcome evaluation are written in terms of behavioral performance expected in individuals and families.

A review of the nursing, management, community health, and community mental health literature revealed a paucity of instruments to measure goal attainment. This provided the impetus for the project undertaken during a 2–year continuing education program sponsored by the University of Maryland and the Division of Nursing, Special Projects Branch. The primary purpose to be achieved in this project was to develop an instrument that could be used to measure goal attainment in nursing situations. Since a goal-oriented nursing record was proposed to implement goal setting and goal attainment (King, 1981), data from the use of this instrument would provide documentation of nursing care in the permanent record of the patient, thus supplying the information that determines the effectiveness of nursing care.

A second purpose was to develop, from a nursing perspective, a reliable and valid tool that could be used to conduct research related to a theory of goal attainment in nursing situations.

The conceptual framework for nursing was a theory of goal attainment (King, 1981). This theory for nursing identified both process and outcome variables. Process variables included mutual goal setting and nurse and patient verbal and nonverbal communication behaviors relevant in the interactions that lead to transactions. Outcome variables were the goals attained by patients as a result of mutual goal setting and transactions made. In an initial study to identify the process of nurse–patient interactions that lead to transactions and goals, direct observations of nurse–patient interactions in the natural environment of a hospital unit provided data for analysis. Outcomes thus represented evidence-based practice. This small study resulted in a classification system to study interactions that lead to transactions.

In designing an instrument to measure goal attainment, one problem in nursing was addressed. Nurses have always set goals for nursing care but have not always stated them in terms of expected patient performance behavior that is observable and/or measurable. Mager's (1965) framework was selected for writing goals in terms of patient performance. The goal statements were based on the functional abilities assessment scales that were part of this project.

PROCEDURES FOR DEVELOPMENT

Several factors are considered essential in the development of a criterion-referenced instrument. Waltz and associates (1984) noted "the primary goal of criterion-referenced measurement is to accurately determine the status of some objects in terms of a well-defined domain" (p. 164). A clear definition of the content domain was essential in developing the instrument.

The content domain for this criterion-referenced tool can be described as functional abilities of individuals and as goal attainment behaviors. Functional abilities were defined more specifically as the physical ability of individuals to perform activities of daily living and the behavioral response of individuals to the performance of these activities. Goal attainment was defined as mutual goal setting by nurse and patient on the basis of data from the assessment of functional abilities and from the nurse–patient interactions in which they share information about the presenting conditions and/or problems to be solved.

Subsequent to defining the content domain of the criterion-referenced measure, a homogeneous collection of items was written that accurately assess the content domain. A distinguishing feature of a criterion-referenced measure is that it is based on a specified domain rather than on a specified population or group. Performance standards that defined the domain status were determined. Evaluation of the performance of individuals relative to these standards determined a person's status.

The criterion-referenced measure was designed to measure outcomes, that is, the ability of individuals to perform activities of daily living. The domain objectives were

1. To assess the physical ability of individuals to perform activities of daily living related to personal hygiene, movement, and human interaction
2. To assess the behavioral response of individuals in the performance of these activities
3. To select a goal and to measure goal attainment in performing these activities

A criterion-referenced instrument was constructed that consisted of three scales representing the domain objectives: physical abilities, behavioral response, and goals. Each scale was composed of three subscales: personal hygiene, movement, and human interaction. Multiple items within each subscale were written. The personal hygiene subscale consisted of eight items representative of essential tasks in performing actions related to hygiene. Six items were written that were representative of the movement subscale. The human interaction subscale included 12 items representative of sensory perceptions, verbal and nonverbal communication, and interactions and transactions (see Appendix to this chapter).

DESCRIPTION

A clear specification of the behaviors to be measured was characterized by an essential and behavioral response of the patient in a nursing situation. Data from these assessment scales were used to identify a feasible goal for patients and to measure their attainment of the goal.

Each of the three scales was developed to clearly describe the behaviors of patients. The goal scale was written to specify outcomes that are the performance standards to be attained by patients (see Appendix).

Several standards were identified to create the items in the personal hygiene, movement, and human interaction subscales. First, a decision was made to construct a 4–point scale. Second, items in each of the subscales were developed to assess a range of behaviors from dependence to independence in the performance of activities of daily living. Third, consistency in the terms used to indicate specific behaviors at each level of performance was considered to be essential in item writing. Fourth, a sufficient number of items within each subscale was developed to sample the essential behaviors expected in patients' performance of activities of daily living. This instrument was designed to be used by registered professional nurses. The following example illustrates the general description for a measure of *physical ability* to perform mouth care: "Brushes teeth/dentures, without assistance"; the general description for a measure of *behavioral response* to performing mouth care: "Assumes responsibility for daily oral hygiene"; and the general description for a measure of *goal attainment*: "Given the equipment, health reasons for mouth care, and a demonstration of techniques, patient performs mouth care a minimum of two times a day."

Sample Item

The first draft of the instrument was analyzed by 10 graduate students in clinical nursing of adults. Suggestions for clarity were given and several items were revised, but none were discarded. The next step in the process was to write clear directions for using the instrument and for scoring.

ADMINISTRATION AND SCORING

Using the assessment data, nurses set goals with patients and measure goal attainment by scoring the differences between goals set and goals attained. The initial assessment takes about 15 minutes and serves as baseline data for comparison with future assessments. Direct observations of patients' ability to perform the functions of daily activities are required to assess patients.

Only registered professional nurses are responsible for using the instrument for goal setting and for measuring goal attainment. This is a professional nursing function within which decisions are made for nursing care. This criterion-referenced instrument measures each individual's attainment of goals. Data from the assessment scales and from the goal attainment scale are placed on the permanent patient record to be used by professional nurses in planning, implementing, and evaluating effectiveness of care. The results are used to determine status of patients based on performance standards specified in the domain.

The 4–point scale contains items that are ordered from dependence to independence. Definitions for functional dependence and independence are as follows:

1. Completely dependent; patient needs help with the activity
2. Requires assistance by caregiver or mechanical aid in performance of the activity
3. Requires supervision; patient is independent of caregiver but needs monitoring of performance of activity
4. Independent of caregiver; patient can perform the activity with or without mechanical aids

If the nurse gives the patient a score of 1 on physical ability to brush teeth, the goal to be attained may be set at 3. The highest goal attainment score for anyone is 4. If the goal is set at 3 and the patient attains 3, this is equal to 0, or congruence between goal set and goal attained. The score for patients can range from –3 to +3. For example, if the goal is set at 3 and the patient achieves 1, the expected goal is not attained and a score of minus 2 is recorded. If the goal is set at 1 and the patient achieves 4, then the score is +3 and exceeds expected performance. The standard score is set for each individual on a scale of 1 to 4; for example, 1 equals dependence in functioning, and 4 equals independence in functioning. In some instances a percentage score may be used in a criterion-referenced instrument as a measure of absolute performance. The formula to convert a raw score to a percentage score is:

$$\text{Percentage Score} = \frac{\text{subject's raw score on measure}}{\text{maximum possible raw score}} \times 100$$

If the raw score on goal attainment is 3, then performance score is 3/4 × 100, or 75%.

RELIABILITY AND VALIDITY

Validity

The initial draft of the instrument was revised to be consistent with Mager's (1965) suggestions for writing objectives that are measurable. Each goal scale should contain three elements: (1) describe the respondent (the patient), (2) describe the behavior the respondent will demonstrate when the goal is achieved, (3) describe the conditions under which the respondent demonstrates goal attainment.

In determining content validity each item represents a measure of the content domain. The judgment of two content specialists in nursing was used to assess the validity of the items within three major categories of functional abilities related to personal hygiene, movement, and human interaction. The two judges were given the domain objectives, the set of items, and a form for recording their rating of the relevance of each item to a domain. For example, 1 = not relevant; 2 = somewhat relevant; 3 = quite relevant; 4 = very relevant. Content validity is the proportion of items rated as quite/very relevant (3 or 4) by both judges. A content validity index (CVI) of .88 was obtained.

Content validity was also achieved in the systematic way the tool was developed. A content analysis was done on four tools currently used to assess functional abilities. A category system was developed from this analysis, resulting in the three subscales. The categories also represented elements in King's theory of goal attainment and definition of health (King, 1981).

The measurement literature indicated that terms used to describe validity for criterion-referenced measures were different than those used for norm-referenced measures. For example, Popham (1978) used the terms *descriptive* and *functional validity*. He noted that descriptive validity was related to content validity. When items are congruent with domain objectives, congruency percentages of 90 or higher are satisfactory. He described functional validity as the accuracy with which a criterion-referenced measure satisfies the purpose for its use. This is like criterion-related validity if accurate predictions can be made.

Another type of validity for criterion-referenced measures is decision validity, in which appropriate decisions result from scores on a measure. Data from the two assessment scales were used to make decisions about goal setting and goal attainment. This instrument has content validity and decision validity.

Reliability

Estimates of interrater reliability were determined. Two nurses with master of science degrees in nursing volunteered to use the instrument to assess 20 patients in a nursing home setting. These nurses were equally familiar with the patients. Since there was minimal variability in this homogeneous group of patients, percentage of interrater agreement was determined rather than product-moment correlations. The interrater agreement for the total score was 85%. Interrater agreement on each of three subscales was 83% for physical ability, 84% for behavior response, and 87% for goal attainment. Percentage of agreement was obtained for each item and ranged from 63% to 100%.

A second sample of 20 patients in a critical care unit of a large metropolitan hospital was assessed by two nurses with BSN degrees. Product-moment correlation coefficients of interrater reliability were determined for this sample, which was more heterogeneous than the nursing home sample. Estimates of interrater reliability for the instrument were .99 for the three scales and for the three subscales:

1. Physical ability: personal hygiene, .99; movement, .95; and human interaction, .92.
2. Behavior response: personal hygiene, .99; movement, .97; and human interaction, .92.
3. Goal attainment: personal hygiene, .99; movement, .97; and human interaction, .92.

Item correlations ranged from .70 to 1.00 with sleep and written communication below .70 (.54 and .68).

Interscale relationships were determined between physical ability and behavior response, between physical ability and goal attainment, and between behavior response and goal attainment. Correlations between the physical scale and the behavior scale on the three subscales were as follows: personal hygiene, .99; movement, .98; and human interaction, 1.00. Correlations between the physical scale and the goal scale were as follows: personal hygiene, .99; movement, .99; and human interaction, 1.00. Correlations between the behavior and the goal scale were as follows: personal-hygiene, .99; movement, .99; human interaction, 1.00. Because the interscale correlations yielded by the two nurses were not significantly different, the interscale correlations represent the averages of the correlations from the two nurses.

CONCLUSIONS AND RECOMMENDATIONS

The purpose of this project has been achieved. This instrument, which has a CVI of .88 and reliability of .99, provides a tool for nurses to assess functional abilities of patients, to make decisions about goal setting with and for patients, and to measure goal attainment. Goals set and goals attained provide a measure of effectiveness of care, which represents evidence-based nursing practice. The reliability and validity of this instrument augur well for its use in nursing research that tests hypotheses generated from King's theory of goal attainment.

One of the results of developing this criterion-referenced measure was the demonstration of a need to develop many more tools for use in nursing research and practice. This instrument was limited to measurement of functional abilities and goal attainment of individuals within three subscales of personal hygiene, movement, and human interaction. The format can be used to develop instruments to measure goal attainment in other areas of nursing practice.

REFERENCES

King, I. M. (1981). *A theory for nursing: Systems, concepts and process.* New York: Wiley.

King, I. M. (1988). Measuring Health Goal Attainment in patients. In C. F. Waltz & O. L. Strickland (Eds.), *Measurement of nursing outcomes* (pp. 109–127). New York: Springer Publishing Co.

Mager, R. R. (1965). *Preparing instructional objectives.* Palo Alto, CA: Fearon.

Popham, W. J. (1978). *Criterion-referenced measurement.* Englewood, NJ: Prentice Hall.

Waltz, C., Strickland, O., & Lenz, E. (1984). *Measurement in nursing research.* Philadelphia: Davis.

APPENDIX: A Criterion-Referenced Measure of Goal Attainment:
Assessment of Functional Abilities and Goal Attainment Scales

Scale 1: Physical ability to perform activity	Scale 2: Behavior response to perform activity	Scale 3: Goal to be attained by patient

PERSONAL HYGIENE

Mouth care

Unable to brush teeth/ dentures	Rejects assistance in brushing teeth/ dentures	Oral hygiene provided by caregiver with demonstration of technique and health reasons for mouth care given to patient
Requires assistance with equipment and brushing	Tolerates assistance with mouth care	Demonstrates adequate mouth care under supervision of caregiver
Requires supervision with equipment and brushing teeth/ dentures	Seeks assistance in brushing teeth/ dentures	Demonstrates proper technique in perform-ing mouth care once a day
Brushes teeth/dentures without assistance	Assumes responsibility for oral hygiene	Uses appropriate technique in perform-ing mouth care a minimum of two times a day

Bathing

Unable to bathe self	Rejects assistance with complete bath	Permits caregiver to give bath
Requires assistance with bathing except for hands and face	Tolerates assistance in bathing but washes face and hands	Permits caregiver to bathe back, legs, and torso
Requires supervision when bathing self	Seeks assistance in bathing self	Bathes self when assisted into tub/ shower
Bathes self without assistance	Assumes responsibility for daily bath	Takes shower/bath safely once a day without assistance

Eating

Unable to feed self	Rejects assistance with eating and drinking	Permits caregiver to feed him/her

APPENDIX *(continued)*

Scale 1: Physical ability to perform activity	Scale 2: Behavior response to perform activity	Scale 3: Goal to be attained by patient
Requires assistance with eating and drinking	Tolerates assistance with eating and drinking	Asks to select food and liquids and eats and drinks with assistance
Requires supervision when eating and drinking	Seeks assistance when eating and drinking	Given food selected by patient, eats slowly and in small amounts 4 times a day
Eats and drinks without assistance	Assumes responsibility for eating and drinking without assistance	Selects appropriate food, eats and drinks 3 times a day without assistance

Dressing

Unable to dress self	Rejects assistance in dressing	Permits caregiver to dress him/her
Requires assistance with dressing	Tolerates assistance in dressing	Assists caregiver in dressing self
Requires supervision when dressing self	Seeks assistance in dressing self	Dresses self with supervision 50% of the time
Dresses self without assistance	Assumes responsibility for dressing self each day	Dresses self without assistance 100% of the time

Grooming

Unable to perform grooming activities	Refuses to perform grooming activities	Permits caregiver to perform grooming activities
Requires assistance with grooming activities	Tolerates assistance with grooming	Assists caregiver with grooming
Requires supervision with grooming activities	Seeks assistance with grooming activities	Performs grooming with supervision 5% of the time
Performs grooming activities without assistance	Assumes responsibility for grooming activities	Performs basic grooming activities 100% of the time

Bladder

Unable to pass urine	Rejects chemical/mechanical aids	Accepts use of chemical/mechanical aids to pass urine
Requires assistance in use of chemical/mechanical aids to pass urine	Tolerates assistance in use of chemical/mechanical aids	Cooperates with caregiver in use of aids

APPENDIX *(continued)*

Scale 1: Physical ability to perform activity	Scale 2: Behavior response to perform activity	Scale 3: Goal to be attained by patient
Requires supervision in use of chemical/mechanical aids to pass urine	Seeks assistance in use of chemical/mechanical aids	Seeks supervision in use of aids
Passes urine with or without chemical/mechanical aids	Assumes responsibility for using aids when necessary	Maintains adequate urinary elimination daily with or without aids

Bowels

Unable to have bowel movement	Refuses chemical/mechanical aids	Accepts use of aids
Requires assistance in use of chemical/mechanical aids	Tolerates use of chemical/mechanical aids	Cooperates with caregiver in use of aids
Requires supervision in use of chemical/mechanical aids	Seeks assistance in use of aids	Seeks supervision in selection of aids to use
Defecates with or without assistance of chemical/mechanical aids	Assumes responsibility for using aids when necessary	Maintains adequate bowel elimination with or without aids based on pattern of defecation once a day

Continence

Total incontinence relative to urination/defecation	Unaware of incontinence	Aware of incontinence by verbalizing discomfort
Partial/total incontinence with urination/defecation	Expresses fear and embarrassment due to incontinence	Cooperates with care in planning to control incontinence
Partial/total control by catheter, enemas, or regular toilet times	Seeks assistance in controlling incontinence	Seeks supervision in establishing patterns of elimination to control incontinence
Urination/defecation controlled by self	Assumes responsibility for control of incontinence	Controls incontinence with or without chemical/mechanical aids 100% of the time

MOVEMENT

Walking

Unable to walk	Rejects mechanical or caregiver assistance in trying to walk	Permits caregiver to move legs and arms and sits up in bed

APPENDIX *(continued)*

Scale 1: Physical ability to perform activity	Scale 2: Behavior response to perform activity	Scale 3: Goal to be attained by patient
Requires mechanical or caregiver assistance to walk from bed to chair	Tolerates mechanical or caregiver assistance in walking from bed to chair	Caregiver assists in walking 10 feet
Requires mechanical or caregiver supervision in walking 100 feet	Seeks mechanical or caregiver assistance in walking 100 feet	Walks 100 feet using supportive aids under supervision of caregiver
Walks without caregiver assistance	Walks within physical limits wit mechanical aids	Walks safely with or without mechanical aids

Wheelchair

Unable to transfer to wheelchair from bed	Rejects assistance in transfer from bed to wheelchair	Given a demonstration of techniques for transfer, patient is able to perform arm, leg, and body movement in bed
Requires caregiver or mechanical assistance to transfer from bed to wheelchair and wheelchair to bed	Tolerates assistance in transfer from bed to wheelchair and wheelchair to bed	Demonstrates transfer from bed to wheel-chair and wheelchair to bed with caregiver assistance
Requires supervision to transfer from bed to wheelchair and wheelchair to bed	Seeks assistance in transfer from bed to wheelchair and wheelchair to bed	Transfers safely to and from bed to wheel-chair with caregiver supervision
Transfers safely without assistance from caregiver	Assumes responsibility for transferring safely from bed to wheel-chair and wheelchair to bed	Transfers safely from bed to wheelchair and wheelchair to bed independently 100% of the time

In Bed

Unable to turn, sit up, or get in or out of bed	Rejects assistance in turning and sitting up in bed	Permits caregiver to turn and to sit up in bed
Requires assistance to turn, sit up, and get in or out of bed	Tolerates assistance in turning and sitting up in bed	Demonstrates tech-niques in turning and sitting up in bed with caregiver assistance

APPENDIX *(continued)*

Scale 1: Physical ability to perform activity	Scale 2: Behavior response to perform activity	Scale 3: Goal to be attained by patient
Requires supervision in getting in and out of bed	Seeks assistance in getting in and out of bed	Moves in and out of bed with caregiver assistance
Moves in and out of bed with or without mechanical support	Assumes responsibility within physical limits to move in and out of bed	Moves safely in and out of bed without caregiver assistance

Exercises

Unable to exercise	Rejects assistance in exercising	Permits 15 minutes of passive exercise a day
Requires complete assistance in active exercises	Tolerates passive exercises and assistance with active exercises	Demonstrates active exercises in arms and legs for 10 minutes a day
Requires partial assistance in active exercise	Seeks assistance in active exercise	Demonstrates active exercise in extremities in walking 15 minutes a day
Exercises without caregiver assistance	Assumes responsibility for daily exercises	Exercises consistently in moderation a minimum of 15 minutes a day

Range of Motion

Unable to move extremities	Rejects assistance to move legs and arms	Permits caregiver to put extremities through full range of motion
Requires caregiver assistance to move legs and arms	Tolerates assistance in moving legs and arms	Demonstrates partial range of motion with assistance twice a day
Requires caregiver to supervise movement of legs and arms	Seeks assistance of caregiver in moving legs or arms	Demonstrates full range of motion in extremities with assistance twice a day
Moves legs and arms independently	Expresses satisfaction in ability to move extremities	Demonstrates full range of motion in extremities without assistance twice a day

Sleep

Unable to sleep at night	Rejects all forms of assistance by caregiver	Verbalizes long-term use and effect of sleeping pills

APPENDIX *(continued)*

Scale 1: Physical ability to perform activity	Scale 2: Behavior response to perform activity	Scale 3: Goal to be attained by patient
Requires chemical assistance to sleep at night	Tolerates assistance with relaxation techniques to accompany use of medications	Demonstrates to caregiver the use of two relaxation techniques
Requires supervision with relaxation techniques	Seeks assistance to use relaxation techniques	Demonstrates to caregiver use of two relaxation techniques learned from pamphlets, AV material, and caregiver's demonstration
Able to sleep without chemical assistance	Expresses satisfaction in ability to sleep without chemical assistance	Performs relaxation technique each evening prior to bedtime

HUMAN INTERACTION

Consciousness

Unable to arouse (comatose)	No response to painful or noxious stimuli	Demonstrates no response to painful or noxious stimuli
Requires use of strong verbal and tactile stimuli (stuporous or semiconscious)	Responds lucidly to verbal stimuli followed by irrational response	Demonstrates lucid response to verbal stimuli 50% of the time
Requires assistance with complex mental activity (confused)	Responds slowly to sensory stimuli and simple mental activity; oriented to time, place, and some persons	Demonstrates slow response during interactions with individuals in environment 100% of the time
Able to interact in time and place with individuals	Responds to sensory stimuli, oriented to time, place, and persons	Demonstrates orientation to time, place, persons through appropriate interactions with individuals 100% of the time

Hearing

Unable to hear or read lips	No response and unable to read lips	Demonstrates ability to place hearing aid in ear with 100% accuracy

APPENDIX *(continued)*

Scale 1: Physical ability to perform activity	Scale 2: Behavior response to perform activity	Scale 3: Goal to be attained by patient
Requires complete assistance with use of mechanical aid	Tolerates mechanical aid	Demonstrates ability to adjust hearing aid to environment with 100% accuracy
Requires partial assistance with use of mechanical aid	Seeks assistance if necessary	Demonstrates use of hearing aid with 100% accuracy
Can distinguish sounds and hear conversation with or without mechanical aid	Expresses satisfaction in use of mechanical aid	Demonstrates ability to engage in normal conversations with hearing aid with 100% accuracy

Vision

Unable to see without glasses	Refuses help from caregivers in movement in the environment and with personal hygiene	Accepts caregiver's assistance with activities of daily living
Requires assistance in the environment without glasses	Tolerates partial assistance with personal hygiene and movement in limited environment	Performs personal hygiene and moves about room with assistance of caregiver
Requires supervision to get used to glasses in moving around in the room	Tolerates glasses and moves cautiously in limited environment	Demonstrates use of special glasses and cares for self without assistance
Performs activities of daily living independently and moves around in familiar surroundings with glasses	Expresses satisfaction in taking walks in the environment	Performs activities of daily living and moves around in familiar surroundings without assistance

Smell

Unable to detect noxious odors	Rejects help in detecting differences in odors	Permits caregiver to present a variety of odors to learn differences
Requires assistance to differentiate one odor from another	Tolerates assistance in differentiating between normal odors and harmful odors	Practices differentiating pleasant from harmful odors

APPENDIX *(continued)*

Scale 1: Physical ability to perform activity	Scale 2: Behavior response to perform activity	Scale 3: Goal to be attained by patient
Requires supervision to differentiate one odor from another	Seeks feedback and reinforcement in differentiating odors	Demonstrates discrimination of odors with 70% accuracy
Discriminates odors without assistance	Responds slowly in differentiating odors	Demonstrates discrimination of odors with 100% accuracy

Taste

Unable to distinguish between sweet, sour, salty, bitter tastes and temperatures	Rejects help to distinguish different taste sensations	Tastes different kinds of foods and liquids to try to distinguish between various taste sensations and temperatures
Requires assistance to determine differences in taste sensations and temperatures	Tolerates assistance in distinguishing taste sensations and temperatures	Demonstrates differences between sweet, sour, salty, bitter foods, and hot and cold liquids with 50% accuracy
Requires supervision in differentiating taste sensations and temperatures	Seeks assistance in distinguishing taste sensations and temperature	Demonstrates with 75% accuracy differences between sweet, sour, salty, bitter foods, and hot and cold
Differentiates tastes and temperature without assistance	Verbalizes satisfaction in distinguishing tastes and temperatures	Demonstrates with 100% accuracy differences between sweet, sour, salty, bitter foods, and hot and cold

Touch

Unable to detect sensation of light touch, heat, or cold	Rejects assistance in detecting sensation of light touch, heat, or cold	With assistance from caregiver practices touching objects and describing cutaneous sensation
Requires assistance to sense light touch, heat, and cold	Tolerates assistance in differentiating between light touch, heat, and cold	Demonstrates discrimination between sensations of light touch, heat, and cold with 50% accuracy
Requires supervision with objects that are hot or cold	Seeks assistance in differentiating between heat and cold	Demonstrates with 75% accuracy discrimination between sensations of light touch, heat and cold

APPENDIX *(continued)*

Scale 1: Physical ability to perform activity	Scale 2: Behavior response to perform activity	Scale 3: Goal to be attained by patient
Discriminates between sensations of light touch, heat, and cold	Expresses satisfaction in ability to differentiate cutaneous sensations	Demonstrates with 100% accuracy discrimination between cutaneous sensations of light touch, heat and cold

Communication, Verbal

Unable to speak	Rejects assistance in using words	Demonstrates use of simple words correctly 100% of time
Speaks words slowly	Tolerates assistance in using words to communicate to caregiver	Demonstrates use of sentences correctly 100% of time
Speaks sentences slowly with cues from others	Seeks assistance to reinforce use of words in sentences	Demonstrates ability to speak slowly and clearly 100% of the time
Uses sentences appropriately when interacting with other human beings	Expresses satisfaction in ability to carry on a conversation with others	Demonstrates ability to engage in a conversation with others 100% of the time

Listening

Unable to comprehend spoken words	Rejects assistance by caregiver to repeat messages slowly	Demonstrates comprehension of simple words when spoken slowly and clearly
Responds to spoken messages with assistance from therapist/caregiver	Tolerates spoken messages	Demonstrates comprehension of spoken sentences 100% of time when delivered slowly and clearly
Responds to spoken messages with minimal assistance from therapist/caregiver	Seeks reinforcement that message is understood	Demonstrates comprehension of verbal messages 100% of time
Comprehends spoken messages	Expresses pleasure in listening to persons, to TV, and to radio	Demonstrates ability to listen and respond appropriately 100% of time

APPENDIX *(continued)*

Scale 1: Physical ability to perform activity	Scale 2: Behavior response to perform activity	Scale 3: Goal to be attained by patient
Reading		
Unable to read	Refuses to read	Demonstrates ability to read menu and select food
Requires assistance in reading menu	Tolerates assistance with reading menu and instruction for diagnostic tests	Demonstrates ability to read diet instructions 100% of time
Requires supervision in reading about diet and medications	Seeks assistance to understand what is read about diet and medications	Demonstrates ability to read and understand instructions for diagnostic tests, diet, and medications 100% of the time
Able to read magazines and books	Expresses pleasure in reading anything in the environment	Demonstrates ability to read and comprehend articles, books, and directions within educational background with 100% accuracy
Writing		
Unable to write	Rejects assistance in writing simple words	Demonstrates use of pad and pencil to write simple words
Requires assistance in writing words	Tolerates assistance in writing sentences	Demonstrates ability to write clear sentences 100% of time
Requires supervision in writing sentences	Seeks assistance to write clear messages	Demonstrates ability to write clear messages 75% of time
Writes sentences that clearly communicate messages	Expresses satisfaction when written messages are understood by others	Demonstrates ability to communicate clearly in writing 100% of the time
Communication, Nonverbal		
Unable to interact with gestures	Rejects assistance to purposefully interact nonverbally	Uses several meaningful gestures to interact with caregiver

APPENDIX *(continued)*

Scale 1: Physical ability to perform activity	Scale 2: Behavior response to perform activity	Scale 3: Goal to be attained by patient
Requires assistance to use meaningful gestures	Tolerates assistance to use meaningful gestures	Demonstrates use of gestures that clearly communicate 100% of the time
Requires partial assistance with gestures Interacts clearly and appropriately with gestures	Seeks feedback and reinforcement for clear nonverbal interactions Responds with satisfaction when nonverbal gestures communicate messages clearly	Demonstrates clear communication through use of nonverbal techniques 100% of time Interacts clearly with appropriate nonverbal techniques 100% of the time

Transactions (decisions)

Unable to make transactions with caregiver	Rejects participation in decision making about care	Demonstrates beginning acceptance of responsibility for decisions about health status
Requires assistance in decision making that leads to transactions	Tolerates assistance in making decisions	Demonstrates ability to make some decisions that lead to transactions
Requires supervision by caregiver in making transactions that lead to goals	Seeks feedback and reinforcement in decision making that leads to transactions	Demonstrates ability to make transactions that lead to goal attainment 75% of the time
Able to make decisions that lead to transactions and goal attainment	Expresses satisfaction with transactions that lead to goal attainment	Makes transactions with relevant others that lead to goal attainment 100% of the time

2

Multidimensional Functional Assessment of the Elderly: The Iowa Self-Assessment Inventory

Woodrow W. Morris and Kathleen C. Buckwalter

This chapter presents the Iowa Self-Assessment Inventory (ISAI), a self-administered multidimensional functional assessment questionnaire designed for use with older adults.

PURPOSE

The Iowa Self-Assessment Inventory (ISAI) was designed as a multidimensional functional assessment measure, which can be used when planning for and providing services to older persons. Such assessment should furnish at least an aggregate measure of cognitive, affective, social, and activities of daily living functioning (Kane & Kane, 1981).

The need for multidimensional functional assessment relates to the growing range of needs of older persons as time goes on. With multiple diagnoses, targeting the most appropriate support services becomes increasingly complex. Comprehensive assessment can help formulate treatment plans, aid in the casework process, assist with teaching and training of care providers, and facilitate planning of needed facilities and services.

Morris and Boutelle (1985) examined the feasibility of a self-administered assessment instrument. Their study suggested that the logical next step would be the development of a psychometrically constructed inventory that could be easily and quickly scored, that would provide information basic to understanding the needs and status of individuals, and could be used for surveys of large groups of older persons. The ISAI addresses these needs.

CONCEPTUAL BASIS OF THE IOWA
SELF-ASSESSMENT INVENTORY

The conceptual basis of the ISAI was derived from the Multidimensional Functional Assessment Questionnaire (MFAQ) (Duke University, 1978). It is also referred to as the OARS methodology, the acronym being taken from Duke's Older American Resources and Services Program. The OARS methodology led to the conceptualization of a basic model that is not only useful for approaching the specific options in long-term care, but also issues related to program evaluation and resource allocation decisions. The element of the model that supported the development of the ISAI is that of providing a procedure for measuring functional status of individuals and a related scheme for classifying individuals with similar status (equivalence classes). Surveys of the literature and clinical experiences indicated that information was necessary on five dimensions—social resources, economic resources, mental health, physical health, and activities of daily living (ADL) if a comprehensive overview of individual functioning is to be obtained (Fillenbaum, 1988). Certain information was considered basic to a determination of level of functioning:

Social resources—quantity and quality of relationships with friends and family; availability of care in time of need
Economic resources—adequacy of income and physical/environmental resources
Mental health—extent of psychiatric well-being and presence of organicity
Physical health—presence of physical disorders, participation in physical activities
Activities of daily living (ADL)—capacity to perform various instrumental and physical (bodily care) tasks that permit individuals to live independently

The ISAI builds upon the OARS, but is distinct from it because it is designed to be self-administered, and it takes much less time to complete (approximately 10 to 20 minutes), whereas the OARS requires an interview that takes from 45 minutes to more than an hour to administer. Therefore, the ISAI is especially suited for brief clinical self-assessments and for use in large-scale surveys without the need for face-to-face data collection.

PROCEDURES FOR DEVELOPMENT

The ISAI was originally developed to measure the five dimensions of the OARS methodology (Fillenbaum, 1988): (1) social resources, (2) economic resources, (3) mental health status, (4) physical health status, and

(5) ability to carry on the activities of daily living. Items were added to measure a sixth dimension, cognitive status (Morris & Buckwalter, 1988). Originally, twenty items were used to measure each dimension for a total of 120 items.

A study by Morris and associates (1989) evaluated the subscale reliabilities and presented evidence related to the validity of the scales in a large sample of 1,153 elderly persons. These investigators examined the subscale reliabilities of the ISAI, which ranged from .74 to .86, and presented evidence related to the validity and relative independence of the scales in a large sample of elderly persons. The conclusions drawn from this study noted acceptable reliabilities for each of the six subscales. The moderate intercorrelations among the scales (.10 to .40) suggested that the scales were assessing the constructs with very little redundancy and overlap. Finally, the relationships between the scales and the demographic variables were generally consistent with expected scale sensitivities.

Subsequent analyses of the factor structure of this 120–item instrument revealed four viable factors: (1) economic resources, (2) physical health, (3) cognitive status, and (4) a factor labeled *mobility* which was related to both social activities and activities of daily living (Morris et al., 1990). Because the areas of social support and mental health were considered important aspects of adaptation in the later years, a number of additional items related to these dimensions were added and tested. Analyses of this revised ISAI revealed three relatively strong scales related to anxiety/depression, alienation (trusting others), and social support. The four original dimensions also retained their identity (Morris et al., 1990). The factor analytic result, however, which supported a seven-factor instrument was based on two different analyses and two different instruments.

As a result of these studies, the current version of the ISAI presented here contains 56 items designed to measure seven dimensions: economic resources, physical health, cognitive status, mobility, emotional balance, trusting others, and social support. The remainder of this report addresses analyses of this latest version of the ISAI in which all 56 items were administered to a single sample of 484 elderly respondents in a predominately rural and small-town Midwestern area.

DESCRIPTION

The seven scales comprising the inventory are arranged in cyclic form as follows: every seventh item, beginning with number one, is an economic resource item; anxiety/depression items make up the next pattern, then physical health items, trusting others items, mobility items, cognitive status items, and, finally, social support items. There are eight items in each of the following dimensions: economic resources, physical health, cognitive status, mobility, emotional balance, trusting others, and social support.

All of the items are posed in the same format, to which responses are given in terms of how true the statement is about them, answered on a 4-point scale: *True, More often true than not, More often false than not, and False.*. The inventory may be scored manually or by computer. Ratings that are considered to be favorable, positive, or healthy are assigned a score of 4, whereas those of an opposite nature are scored 1, with intermediate scores of 3 and 2. Keeping in mind that the ratings of the items in the inventory are the respondents' perceptions of their status with respect to the several areas measured by the scales, scores are defined as follows:

The Economic Resources Scale (ER)—High scores on this scale are obtained by those who perceive their income and assets as adequate and, therefore, have no need for outside financial help, and do not participate in programs designed to supplement one's income. Those who perceive their economic status to be inadequate would obtain low scores on this scale.

The Emotional Balance Scale (EB)—Those with high scores on this scale perceive themselves as relatively worry free, more or less calm, sleep well, and enjoy tranquil lives. Low scores indicate the opposite.

The Physical Health Status Scale (PH)—High scores on this scale suggest the individual who professes excellent health, seldom sees a doctor, and takes few prescribed medications. Those with low scores indicate they have physical illnesses or disabilities, have more health problems than others, and that their ability to carry on activities of daily living has declined over recent years.

The Trusting Others Scale (TO)—Individuals scoring high on this scale are those who believe that they have good, trustworthy friends, are friendly toward others, and are generally amiable and affable in their interpersonal relationships. Low scores indicate that they question the motives of others and believe others are against them. They feel alienated from others.

The Mobility Scale (MO)—High scores on this scale are obtained by those who are mobile enough to carry on the activities of daily living, are able to get out to visit friends and relatives, and can participate in other social activities. Low scores represent the lack of such mobility.

The Cognitive Status Scale (CS)—Those who score high on this scale perceive themselves as intellectually intact, possessing good memories, orientations, and a continued ability to learn. Individuals with low scores tend to report that they have trouble remembering things, forget appointments, and suffer a low attention span.

The Social Support Scale (SS)—High scores on this scale suggest that the respondents believe they live in a comfortable social environment, peopled with friends and relatives with whom they enjoy close relationships. Low scores indicate that they perceive a less supportive social environment.

ADMINISTRATION AND SCORING

Administration of the ISAI may be to individuals or in a group setting. (A copy of the ISAI is attached; see Appendix to this chapter) In either setting, the following instructions may be used:

Tell respondents, "The purpose of this inventory is to determine how you feel about your resources, statuses, abilities, and needs. Knowing these, we hope to be able to respond to your needs and help you obtain necessary resources." Answer any questions the person(s) may have and distribute the ISAI booklet.

Read the instructions as the subjects follow along. Answer questions and, if there are none ask the individual(s) to proceed to complete the form stressing the importance of answering every item.

Scoring of completed forms is accomplished according to the key provided in Table 2.1.

All the item ratings are scored on a four-point scale according to the key in the table. An "R" (Reversal) item is one in which the rating should be reversed: thus, a rating of 4 would be recorded as 1, a rating of 2 would be recorded as 3, and so on. Items designated as "S" (Same) would be recorded as rated. A scale score is obtained by adding these adjusted scores. Since there are 8 statements in each scale, the maximum score

TABLE 2.1 Scoring Key and Manual Scoring Form

Scales	Items								Scores
Economic Resources	1R	8R	15R	22S	29R	36S	43R	50S	
Emotional Balance	2S	9S	16S	23S	30S	37S	44S	51S	
Physical Health	3R	10S	17R	24R	31S	38R	45S	52R	
Trusting Others	4S	11S	18S	25S	32S	39S	46S	53S	
Mobility	5S	12R	19R	26S	33S	40R	47R	54R	
Cognitive Status	6S	13S	20S	27S	34S	41S	48R	55S	
Social Support	7S	14S	21R	28S	35S	42R	49S	56S	

would be 32 and the lowest possible score would be 8. The higher the score, the more positive the assessment. In summary, follow the directions below for scoring the ISAI:

1. Transfer the ratings from the booklet to the scoring form, being sure to reverse all "R" ratings.
2. Total these raw scores for each scale and write the total in the "SCORES" column.
3. Record these scores in the spaces provided at the bottom of the "Profile form." The means and standard deviations of the several scales vary significantly. (To make the scale scores comparable, they were converted to standard scores [T-scores], the distributions of which all have a mean of 50 and a standard deviation of 10.)

On the profile form, write the raw scores in the space provided at the bottom of each column. Then look for that raw score in its column and circle or otherwise mark it. When all of the points are marked, one may connect the points, resulting in the "profile." Average scores are between 40 and 60, one standard deviation above and below the mean of 50. High scores are those above 60, and low scores are those below 40.

RELIABILITY AND VALIDITY EVIDENCE

Exploratory Analyses

Three maximum likelihood (ML) analyses with promax rotation were run on data from 484 elderly respondents specifying six, seven, and eight factors to be extracted. Unweighted least squares (ULS) factor analyses were also performed, but because the results were similar to the ML analyses and because more information is provided with the output from ML runs, the details of the ULS results are not reported here. When six factors were specified the RMS residual was .038. Akaike's information criterion was 3034, and Schwarz's Bayesian criterion was 2305. When seven factors were specified, the RMS residual was .0332, while the Akaike's information criterion was 2854 and Schwarz's criterion was 2319. The RMS residual was .0310 when eight factors were specified, and the Akaike's information criterion and Schwarz's Bayesian criterion were 2756 and 2373, respectively. The results of these analyses suggested that specifying less than six or more than eight factors would not be productive.

Examination of the items for the seven-factor solution provides strong additional support for seven factors. Of the 56 items in the instrument, 53 had their highest loadings on the anticipated dimensions; only nine items had loadings of less than .40.

When only six factors were extracted, the Trusting Others scale did not develop its own identity. Five of the trusting others items tended to load on the same factor as the social support items. The determination of separate scores for the subscales "trusting others" and "social support" can be an important distinction in identifying needed services for the elderly. Symptoms of paranoia (similar to the "trusting others" dimension in the ISAI) are often associated with suspiciousness, hostility, and withdrawal, which can interfere with patient care (Cole, 1987). Eisdorfer (1980) pointed out that paranoia is among the most disturbing symptoms exhibited by older persons experiencing emotional distress and, therefore, warrants a closer inspection; and Harris and Jeste (1988) recommend that assessment of paranoid traits is important because they may characterize late-onset schizophrenia.

Results of the analyses provide strong evidence to support the existence of seven clear and reasonable dimensions in the ISAI. The item loadings also indicate that in all but three cases, each item is measuring the dimension it was designed to measure.

Statistical Characteristics of the Seven Scales

The basic descriptive characteristics for each of the seven scales indicate that they are highly reliable with reliabilities ranging from 0.71 to 0.84. Scale means ranged from 21.03 for the physical health scale to 29.25 for trusting others. Scale intercorrelations ranged from 0.06 to 0.43. These data are very similar to the corresponding statistics reported in Morris et al. (1990). Most of the scale means are within one point of the previous means and the standard deviations are all within six-tenths of a point; the reliabilities differ by no more than .04 from those previously reported. The highest correlations among scales (i.e., those from 0.35 to 0.43) are obtained for variables that would be expected to be somewhat related: trusting others, emotional balance, and social support. The correlations among variables are still small enough, however, to support measuring them with separate scales. For example, the largest disattenuated correlation is only 0.57, occurring between trusting others and social support. This correlation, while demonstrating some overlap, shows that these two scales measure dimensions that are relatively independent.

CONCLUSIONS AND RECOMMENDATIONS

Overall, the analyses discussed in the paper by Gilmer et al. (1991) provide support for the hypothesis that the Iowa Self Assessment Inventory measures the following seven factors in the elderly: (1) economic resources, (2) emotional balance, (3) social support, (4) cognitive status, (5) mobility, (6) physical health, and (7) trusting others.

The exploratory analyses, which specified six, seven, and eight factors, resulted in six- and eight-factor solutions that were not substantively meaningful. In the six-factor solution the items designed to measure trusting others and social support tended to cluster on one difficult-to-interpret factor; when eight factors were extracted, only two items had substantial loadings on the eighth factor. Fifty-three of the 56 items had appropriate loadings on the specific scales they were designed to measure. The LISREL confirmatory factor analysis suggested that the specified seven-factor model was a reasonably good model for explaining the data.

The research demonstrates that the ISAI tends to measure the same seven dimensions that were identified in previous research, which administered two versions of the ISAI to two different samples of elderly. Finally, scale means, standard deviations, reliabilities, and all possible intercorrelations indicate that the ISAI exhibits acceptable reliabilities for each of the seven scales, and the moderate intercorrelations suggest that the scales have little redundancy or overlap. The individual scale means and standard deviations were very similar to those previously reported (Morris et al., 1990).

REFERENCES

Cole, K. (1987). Late life paranoid states. *Geriatric Medicine Today, 6,* 77–86.

Duke University, Center for the Study of Aging and Human Development. (1978). *Multidimensional functional assessment: The OARS methodology* (2nd ed.). Durham, NC: Author.Eisdorfer, C. (1980). Paranoia and schizophrenic disorders in later life. In E. W. Busse and D. G. Blazer (Eds.), *Handbook of geriatric psychiatry* (pp. 329–337). New York: Van Nostrand, Reinhold.

Fillenbaum, G. G. (1988). *Multidimensional functional assessment of older adults: Duke Older American Resources and Services procedures.* Hillsdale, NJ: Erlbaum.

Gilmer, J. S., Cleary, T. A., Lu, Der Fa, Morris, W. W., Buckwalter, K. C., Andrews, P., Boutelle, S., & Hatz, D. L. (1991). The factor structure of the ISAI. *Educational and Psychological Measurement, 51,* 365–375.

Harris, M. J., & Jeste, D. V. (1988). Late onset schizophrenia: An overview. *Schizophrenia Bulletin, 14,* 39–55.

Kane, R. A., & Kane, R. L. (1981). *Assessing the elderly.* Lexington, MA: Lexington Books.

Morris, W., & Boutelle, S. (1985). Multidimensional functional assessment in two modes. *Gerontologist, 25*(6), 638–643.

Morris, W. W., & Buckwalter, K. C. (1988). Functional assessment of the elderly: The Iowa Self-Assessment Inventory. In C. F. Waltz & O. L.

Strickland (Eds), Measurement of nursing outcomes: Vol. 1: Measuring client outcomes (pp.328–351). New York: Springer Publishing Co.

Morris, W. W., Buckwalter, K. C., Cleary, T. A., Gilmer, J. S., Hatz, D. L., & Studer, M. S. (1989). Issues related to the validation of the Iowa Self-Assessment Inventory. *Educational and Psychological Measurement, 49,* 853–861.

Morris, W. W., Buckwalter, K. C., Cleary, T. A., Gilmer, J., Hatz, D. L., & Studer, M. (1990). Refinement of the Iowa Self-Assessment Inventory. *Gerontologist, 30*(2), 243–248.

Morris, W. W., Buckwalter, K. C., Tripp-Reimer, T., Zimmerman, B., Kosmach, S., & Lu, D. F. (1997). Desarrollo perfeccionamiento del Iowa Self-Assessment Inventory. *Revista de Gerontologia, 7*(2), 64–75.

ADDENDUM TO APPENDIX

The ISAI has been translated into Chinese, Dutch, French, Norwegian, Spanish, and Swedish. A Spanish language version was first prepared by Hayden Rios, PhD, then a graduate student in Nursing Education. He is a native of Puerto Rico and intended to use it to obtain data from one or more samples of elderly Puerto Ricans. Due to such language problems as illiteracy and unfamiliarity with the concepts of inventories, Dr. Rios was unable to obtain the data desired. This raised the question, though, of the feasibility of developing a Pan-American Spanish language version of the ISAI. The opportunity presented itself when we became aware of research on just such an attempt by the staff at the University of New Mexico, directed by Dr. Linda Romero.

A Spanish version of the instrument and manual has been published as "Desarrollo perfeccionamiento del Iowa Self Assessment Inventory," by Woodrow W. Morris, Kathleen C. Buckwalter, Toni Tripp-Reimer, Bridget Zimmerman, Steve Kosmach, and Der Fa Lu (1997) *Revista de Gerontologia, 7*(2), 64–75. It was submitted through the good offices of Dr. Antoni Salva, Centre Geriatric Cabanellas and Dr. Ignasi Bolibar, Institut de Recerca Epidemiologica I Clinica, both of Mataro, Barcelona, Spain, The Director is Antonio San Jose of Barcelona, Spain.

THE IOWA SELF ASSESSMENT INVENTORY

BACKGROUND INFORMATION

Name _____ Date _____

Male ___ Female ___ Age on last birthday _____

How far did you go in school? (Check one.)

1.	_____	Grade school or less
2.	_____	Some high school
3.	_____	High school graduate
4.	_____	Business or trade school
5.	_____	Some college
6.	_____	College graduate
7.	_____	Graduate/professional school

What is your race? (Check one.)

1.	_____	White
2.	_____	Hispanic
3.	_____	Asian
4.	_____	Black/African-American
5.	_____	Native American—Indian
6.	_____	Other, please specify

Who lives in your household with you? (Check one.)

1.	_____	No one—I live alone
2.	_____	My spouse lives with me
3.	_____	I live with another relative
4.	_____	Other, please describe

DIRECTIONS

The statements on the following pages are about things that can affect our lives in one way or another. We ask you to describe your own situation using these statements. In this way we hope to understand some of your problems and needs.

Please use the following key in rating each statement:

1—True
2—More often true than not
3—More often false than not
4—False

Please read each statement carefully and then encircle the number corresponding to the answer that best applies to you. We realize that some of the statements may not apply directly to you all the time, but try to do the best you can. Do not worry about giving exactly the right answer; your answer may simply mean the statement is true or false to some degree.

Please try to make an answer to *every* statement.

1 = True
2 = More often true than not
3 = More often false than not
4 = False

	1 2 3 4
1. I have enough money to meet unexpected emergencies	1 2 3 4
2. I sometimes get tense as I think of the day's happenings	1 2 3 4
3. I have no physical disabilities or illnesses at this time	1 2 3 4
4. People secretly say bad things about me	1 2 3 4
5. I need a cane, crutches, walker, or wheelchair to get around	1 2 3 4
6. I have trouble remembering things that happened recently	1 2 3 4
7. There is no one I can turn to in times of stress	1 2 3 4
8. I have enough money to buy those little extras	1 2 3 4
9. I frequently find myself worrying	1 2 3 4
10. I take 3 or more medicines each day	1 2 3 4
11. Friends are disloyal to me behind my back	1 2 3 4
12. I do my own shopping without help	1 2 3 4
13. I forget where I put things	1 2 3 4
14. There is no one I can depend on for aid if I really need it	1 2 3 4
15. I have enough money to meet my regular daily expenses	1 2 3 4
16. I lose sleep over worry	1 2 3 4
17. My overall health is excellent	1 2 3 4
18. I believe I am being plotted against	1 2 3 4
19. I do my own laundry	1 2 3 4
20. I have trouble remembering the names of people I know	1 2 3 4
21. There is someone I can talk to about important decisions	1 2 3 4
22. I need financial help	1 2 3 4
23. I am bothered by thoughts I can't get out of my head	1 2 3 4
24. My health is better than it was 5 years ago	1 2 3 4
25. Someone has it in for me	1 2 3 4
26. Getting around town is a problem for me	1 2 3 4

27. I lose my train of thought in the middle of a
    conversation   1 2 3 4
28. There is no one I feel comfortable talking about
    problems with   1 2 3 4
29. My finances at the present time are excellent   1 2 3 4
30. I am a very nervous person   1 2 3 4
31. My ability to carry on my daily activities is worse than
    it was 5 years ago   1 2 3 4
32. I am sure I am being talked about   1 2 3 4
33. I am not able to prepare my own meals   1 2 3 4
34. Learning new things is harder for me than it used to be 1 2 3 4
35. No one shares my concerns   1 2 3 4
36. My monthly expenses are so high I cannot always pay
    my bills   1 2 3 4
37. I get upset over things   1 2 3 4
38. I have fewer health problems than most older people
    I know   1 2 3 4
39. Someone is controlling my thoughts   1 2 3 4
40. I walk without help   1 2 3 4
41. I forget appointments   1 2 3 4
42. I know people I can depend on to help me if I really
    need it   1 2 3 4
43. I have some savings and/or investments   1 2 3 4
44. I worry over past mistakes   1 2 3 4
45. During the past year I have been so sick I was unable
    to carry on my usual activities   1 2 3 4
46. Strangers look at me critically   1 2 3 4
47. I can visit a friend or relative who lives out of town for
    overnight or longer   1 2 3 4
48. My mind is just as sharp as ever   1 2 3 4
49. If something went wrong, no one would come to my
    assistance
50. I use food stamps   1 2 3 4
51. I have more ups and downs than most people   1 2 3 4
52. During the past year I have been to a doctor fewer
    than 4 times
53. I see things when others do not   1 2 3 4
54. I visit friends in their homes   1 2 3 4
55. I forget to take medicine when I am supposed to   1 2 3 4
56. I do not have close relationships with other people   1 2 3 4

Name_____ Date_____

Gender (circle one)   Female   Male   Age on last birthday_____

T-scores	ER	EB	PH	TO	MO	CS	SS	T-scores
70-								-70
			32			32		
65-		32	31 / 30			31		-65
		31	29			30		
60-	32	30	28 / 27	32	32	29 / 28		-60
	31	29	26		31	27	32	
55-	30	28 / 27	25 / 24		30 / 29	26 / 25	31	-55
	29 / 28	26	23 / 22	31	28	24	30	
50-	27	25 / 24	21	30	27	23	29	-50
	26 / 25	23	20 / 19	29	26 / 25	22 / 21	28	
45-	24	22 / 21	18 / 17		24	20	27	-45
	23 / 22	20	16	28	23 / 22	19 / 18	26	
40-	21	19	15	27	21	17	25	-40
	20	18	14 / 13		20	18		
	19	17	12	26	19	15	24	
35-	18	16	11		18	14	23	-35
	17	15	10	25	17	13	22	
	16	14	9					
30-	15	13	8	24	16 / 15	12 / 11	21	-30
	14 / 13	12		23	14	10	20	
25-	12	11 / 10			13	9		-25
	11 / 10	9		22	12	8	19	
					11		18	
20-	9	8		21	10		17	-20
	8			20	9 / 8		16	
15-							15	-15
				19			14	
10-				18			13	-10
							12	
5-				17			11	-5
				16				
0-				15			10 / 9	-0

Raw Scores								

Iowa Self-Assessment Inventory Profile Form

3

The Levels of Cognitive Functioning Assessment Scale

Jeanne Flannery

This chapter discusses the Levels of Cognitive Functioning Assessment Scale, a measure that assesses traumatic brain injury patients with low responsivity.

PURPOSE

In the United States, 2 million head injuries occur each year. The Brain Injury Association (BIA) estimates that over 373,000 persons sustain head injuries each year severe enough to require hospitalization. Of these, up to 50,000 persons suffer such serious intellectual and behavioral dysfunction that they are unable to resume a normal life (BIA, 1997). Research supports that early intervention has the potential to improve the outcome of brain-injured patients.

Nurses are at the bedside of severely brain-injured patients more than any other member of the rehabilitation team. Nurses have the unique opportunity to observe and evaluate continually the patient's level of cognitive functioning. Therefore, it is imperative that nurses working with patients with acute brain injury have a standardized tool to use to assess the patient's level of cognitive functioning and initiate rehabilitation appropriately. The Levels of Cognitive Functioning Assessment Scale (LOCFAS) is an instrument developed specifically for this purpose (Flannery, 1987, 1993) (see Appendix).

The LOCFAS is multifaceted in that it provides all disciplines a common assessment vocabulary and documentation instrument with which conclusions regarding cognitive functioning can be reached without patients' being required to cooperate. It can then serve as the basis for discussion among disciplines while establishing an appropriate plan of care, as well as assisting the family to understand the stages of the recovery process and how they may participate to enhance recovery. It can further assist the family and staff to recognize events, situations, and timing that can impede the patient's cognitive functioning through re-corded fluctuation in cognition throughout the day (Flannery, 1987, 1993, 1995, 1997, 1998).

CONCEPTUAL BASIS OF THE LEVELS OF COGNITIVE FUNCTIONING SCALE

Based on Neuman's Systems Model (Neuman, 1995), observation is clearly within the parameters of nursing practice. Thus, observation of patient behaviors as output of cognition can be utilized by nurses to provide data about cognitive functioning, and to determine the degree of reaction from the stressor of traumatic brain injury (TBI). Within Neuman's model, the brain's essential features are viewed as being within the basic structure necessary for the existence of the organism. With the stressor of TBI, an individual's lines of resistance may be weakened so as to permit the reaction to reach the basic structure. Severe injury may produce brain death directly, or, through dysfunction, alter other bodily functions to produce death. Effectiveness of secondary interventions may halt this deterioration and save the organism. Tertiary interventions, based on cognitive assessment, are ongoing, with rehabilitation beginning at the time of admission, always striving toward reconstitution, and, at the same time, setting a goal toward achieving the maximum level of wellness.

The conceptual framework that is most congruent with the development of the LOCFAS is Luria's theory of cognitive recovery (Luria, 1973). Although Luria's theory was not used specifically in the development of the Rancho Los Amigos Levels of Cognitive Functioning instrument, from which the LOCFAS is derived, the theoretical assumptions made by Malkmus, Booth, and Kodimer (1980) concerning cognitive assessment and recovery are consistent with Luria's theory of cognitive recovery. Luria theorized that cognitive functioning is a complex system that is not localized in a narrow, circumscribed area of the brain, but takes place through the participation of brain structures working in concert, each making its own particular contribution to the organization of its functional system. He proposed three principal functional units of the brain whose participation is necessary for any type of mental activity. The lowest unit is for regulating tone and waking; the next highest unit is for obtaining, processing, and storing information arriving from the outside world; and the highest level unit is for programming, regulating, and verifying mental activity. Human conscious activity always takes place with the participation of all three units. Each of these basic units is hierarchical in structure and consists of cortical zones, one built upon another. Luria also identified six components of cognition. These components are perception, movement and action, attention, memory, speech, and thinking.

TBI leads to the disruption of multiple aspects of the cognitive systems, including attention, language, higher cortical functions, social behavior and personality, and memory. Luria (1973) theorized that recovery of cognitive functioning after TBI involves dynamic reorganization through retraining. Further, he theorized that recovery of higher cortical functions would not occur without specific rehabilitative therapy. Within his theory, individual assessment of cognitive functioning was necessary to determine the TBI patient's specific strengths and deficits. In order to rehabilitate the patient, the patient's existing strengths and deficits must be assessed so that the regimen for retraining matches these strengths and deficits specifically. Tasks for reorganization must be introduced that are appropriate to the patient's level of cognitive functioning or those tasks will be ineffective for, or even detrimental to, the patient's recovery.

The combination of Neuman's model and Luria's theory of cognitive recovery as a basis for assessing levels of cognitive functioning of TBI patients to enhance cognitive reconstitution (recovery) is depicted in Figure 3.1. Assessment of cognitive functioning provides the nurse with an understanding of the patient's degree of reaction to the stressor and predictive data regarding the reconstitution process. Based on this assessment, the nurse can hypothesize the most appropriate alternatives, or interventions, that will support the patient's strengths and needs and allow for the present cognitive level.

PROCEDURES FOR INSTRUMENT DEVELOPMENT

The LOCFAS was adapted and modified from the Rancho Los Amigos Levels of Cognitive Functioning instrument (Rancho; Malkmus et al., 1980), using only Levels I through V of the eight original levels. These selected lower levels include behaviors more commonly seen in the earliest stages of recovery when the TBI patient is more likely to be in an inpatient acute care setting. The patient at these lower levels of the scale cannot or will not participate in specific neuropsychological assessments, or still is an unpredictable or inefficient participant. Once the patient has accomplished Level V, more sophisticated diagnostic batteries are appropriate for planning the details of the rehabilitation program (Hagen, 1982). However, knowledge of the patient's cognitive functioning while at or below Level V is critical for the development of appropriate care plans for early rehabilitation to maximize recovery. Since admission criteria to rehabilitation facilities require the patient to be at least a Level IV, these patients are likely to be cared for in the acute care facility.

The Rancho is a behavioral rating scale for assessment of cognitive functioning in adults with TBI (Hagen, Malkmus, & Durham, 1979). It was developed by an interdisciplinary team, based on their observations of 1000 patients during recovery following TBI (Malkmus et al., 1980).

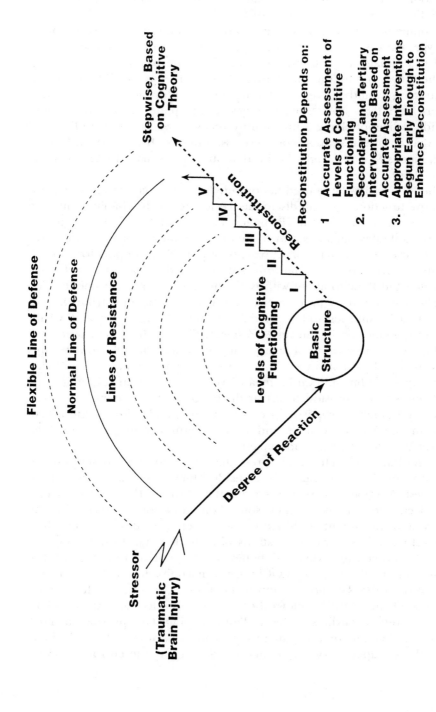

FIGURE 3.1 The combination of Neuman's model and Luria's Theory of Cognitive Recovery: The basis for assessment of levels of cognitive functioning.

The tool provides a way of systematically describing and categorizing the patient's present level of cognitive functioning into one of eight levels. Development of the tool was based on the assumption that observation of the type, nature, and quality of the patient's behavioral responses can be used to estimate the cognitive level at which the patient is functioning. Furthermore, it was theorized that, if recovery was possible, cognitive functioning would be regained following a definable and predictable pattern and that, over time, changes in the patient's behavior would provide indices of changes in cognitive recovery. Subsequent studies have provided empirical support for these assumptions (Brooks, 1984; Craine, 1982; Eames & Wood, 1985; Levin, Benton, & Grossman, 1982; Warren & Peck, 1984).

The Rancho has been used nationwide for more than 25 years to assess cognitive functioning by all disciplines concerned with rehabilitation. The tool is commonly used with TBI patients to provide criteria for admission into rehabilitative facilities and to monitor a patient's progress in recovery. However, the Rancho has a paucity of published support for reliability or validity. Gouvier, Blanton, LaPorte, and Nepomuceno (1987) evaluated the Rancho along with two other assessment instruments. The Rancho was found to have interrater reliabilities ranging from 0.87 to 0.94 (M=0.89) and test–retest reliability of 0.82. Concurrent validity with the Stover-Zeiger Scale (Stover & Zeiger, 1976) was 0.92, and predictive validity from admission to discharge ranged from .57 to .68. However, this study used TBI patients in a rehabilitative facility with a mean of 138 days posttrauma at admission and a mean level of cognitive functioning ranging from 4.8 at admission to 6.1 at discharge on the Rancho. Although these psychometric properties are encouraging, evaluation of the instrument in acute care facilities and with lower-functioning patients (i.e., ≤ Level V) has not been undertaken.

In the Rancho, each level is presented as a behavioral description in narrative form and the rater must decide which level (i.e., which narrative) best describes the patient's present behaviors. However, in reality, the selected level could contain some behaviors not observed with the patient and the patient could exhibit some behaviors described in different-level narratives. Thus, evaluations with the Rancho do not always accurately depict the individual behaviors present at the time of the assessment. To develop the LOCFAS, the narrative for each of the first five levels on the Rancho was transformed into a list of individual behaviors. Use of the LOCFAS allows the evaluator to select only those behaviors observed, regardless of level. Thus, the LOCFAS provides a more accurate reflection of the patient's present behaviors. Table 3.1 shows Level IV as it appears on the Rancho and as it was altered for the LOC-FAS.

TABLE 3.1 Level IV as it Appears on the Original Rancho Los Amigos Levels Of Cognitive Functioning and As It Was Adapted for the Levels of Cognitive Functioning Assessment Scale

RANCHO

IV. *CONFUSED–AGITATED*

Patient is in a heightened state of activity with severely decreased ability to process information. He is detached from the present and responds primarily to his own internal confusion. Behavior is frequently bizarre and non-purposeful relative to his immediate environment. He may cry out or scream out of proportion to stimuli even after removal, may show aggressive behavior, attempt to remove restraints or tubes or crawl out of bed in a purposeful manner. He does not, however, discriminate among persons or objects and is unable to cooperate directly with treatment efforts. Verbalization is frequently incoherent and/or inappropriate to the environment. Confabulation may be present; he may be euphoric or hostile. Thus, gross attention to environment is very short and selective attention is often non-existent. Being unaware of present events, patient lacks short term recall and may be reacting to past events. He is unable to perform self-care (feed, dressing) without maximum assistance. If not disabled physically, he may perform motor activities as in sitting, reaching, and ambulating, but as part of his agitated state and not as a purposeful act or on request necessarily.

LOCFAS

Level IV. CONFUSED-AGITATED
  A. Attention to the Environment: BRIEF
      27. Demonstrates fleeting general attention to surroundings, unable to concentrate
      28. Selective attention may be nonexistent or so brief that it is not acted upon; easily distractible
  B. Response to Stimuli: SPECIFIC, INAPPROPRIATE
      29. May respond consistently to a stimulus, but the response is inappropriate because of internal confusion
      30. May become very agitated or yell in response to a mild stimulus and sustain response after stimulus removed; "sticks" in response; low tolerance for frustration or pain
      31. Responds to presence of devices attachments or anything confining with strong, persistent, purposeful attempt to remove; impatient; demanding
  C. Behavior Status: AGITATED, CONFUSED
      32. In a heightened state of activity related to internal agitation (environment may be quiet and non-stimulating); restless; pacing; rocking; rubbing; moaning
      33. May demonstrate aggressive, hostile behavior; has explosive or unpredictable anger, may be self abusive

TABLE 3.1 *(continued)*

34. May show sudden changes in mood (e.g., crying, laughter, anger, or sleep)
35. Performs overlearned motor activities automatically, but may resist commands to do these same activities, such as "sit up"
D. Ability to Process Information: MINIMAL
  36. Unable to understand or cooperate with treatment efforts; may be combative; resistant to care; will leave areas, if able
E. Ability to Follow Commands: INCONSISTENT
  37. May respond briefly or inconsistently to simple commands when agitation is lessened
F. Awareness of Person (Self):   ORIENTED X1
  38. Is oriented to own name; aware of own body
G. Awareness of Time (Present):   NONE
  39. Unaware of present events; responds primarily to own state of severe confusion
H. Ability to Perform Self Care: MINIMAL
  40. Performs self care activities for brief periods with maximum direction and cueing; cannot focus without redirection
I. Ability to Converse: PRESENT, INAPPROPRIATE
  41. Verbalizes incoherently or with words unrelated to the current situation; talking may be rapid, loud excessive
  42. May confabulate (give incorrect answers to questions about the present from unrelated long-term memory stores); lacks short-term recall
  43. Conversation reflects confusion and memory deficits
J. Ability to Learn New Information: NONE

DESCRIPTION

The current tool (LOCFAS) has evolved, through careful evaluation by cognitive experts, to a behavioral checklist which consists of 61 individual behaviors which are categorized into the first five levels of the Rancho. These behaviors are further sorted into consistent subcategories across all levels. These subcategories include (1) Attention to the Environment, (2) Response to Stimuli, (3) Behavior Status, (4) Ability to Process Information, (5) Ability to Follow Commands, (6) Awareness of Person (self), (7) Awareness of Time, (8) Ability to Perform Self-care, (9) Ability to Converse and (10) Ability to Learn New Information. The number of individual behaviors at each level varies from seven at Level I and II to 18 at Level V. In addition, the number of categories under which these behaviors are grouped also varies. At Level I only three categories are utilized, with no behaviors expected in the others, whereas, at Level V all 10 categories are utilized.

ADMINISTRATION AND SCORING

On the LOCFAS, a grid beside each behavior allows the nurse simply to make a check to indicate the presence of that behavior. Once the checking is completed, visual inspection of the checklist allows the nurse to designate the cognitive level in which most behaviors were observed. This outcome reveals the patient's maximum capacity (i.e., level) at the time of each observation. Repeated use of the instrument also provides a common interdisciplinary language to describe a patient's progress in recovery. More importantly, by identifying the patient's current level of cognitive functioning, the tool can serve as a basis for the development of an appropriate plan of care to facilitate cognitive recovery. It should be noted that the use of the LOCFAS does not provide an interval level assessment of the TBI patient's cognitive functioning. The LOCFAS is a criterion-referenced measure, and the only score a patient receives is Level I, II, III, IV or V. It is the assessment of each specific behavior within the level that is almost as important as the level itself because of the specific interventions that can then be initiated for each. Behaviors present at one level are often replaced by very different behaviors at a higher level. For example, a Level I patient is in the deepest possible stage of coma. Seven behaviors are assessed on the LOCFAS for this level and include items such as unresponsive to auditory, tactile, and painful stimuli. In contrast, a Level IV patient is no longer comatose, but remains disoriented to time and place. He or she can respond to simple commands but is unable to learn new tasks. Seventeen behaviors are included at this level (See Table 3.1 for specific Level IV behaviors).

RELIABILITY AND VALIDITY EVIDENCE

Beginning with studies published in 1993 and continuing through 1998, construct, content, criterion-related, concurrent, and predictive validity have been evaluated. Additionally, intrarater, interrater, and test-retest reliability were tested with a variety of different participants. Table 3.2 summarizes the findings from these studies. Currently, the tool is being used in a 700–bed medical center as an expectation for all nurse employees caring for patients with altered cognitive functioning. Mandatory in-service programs have been conducted by the researcher, including the use of the nursing management plan for each level, and all have been incorporated into the Standards of Care. Additionally, the tool has been widely requested throughout the United States, as well as in a variety of foreign countries. No findings have been reported to the researcher from its use in this 700-bed medical center.

TABLE 3.2 Studies Supporting the Reliability and Validity of LOCFAS

Study citation	Sample and characteristics	Reliability evidence	Validity evidence
Flannery, J. (1993). Psychometric properties of a cognitive functioning scale for TBI patients. *Western Journal of Nursing Research, 15*, 465–482	Study I 13 national and international experts in the area of cognitive theory		*Construct validity:* 70.6% of the behaviors from LOCFAS were categorized in the correct sequential level by more than half the experts Content Validity: 94% of the behaviors from LOCFAS were selected as a behavior critical to categorizing cognitive functioning by more than half the experts
	Study II 18 local and regional experts in cognitive functioning, assessment , and rehabilitation evaluated written vignettes of TBI patients using LOCFAS	*Interrater:* coefficient kappa = 1.00 for agreement among levels and .871 for agreement among items	
	Study III 237 nurses and senior nursing students evaluated written vignettes of TBI patients using LOCFAS	*Interrater:* coefficient kappa = .98 for levels and .925 for items	

TABLE 3.2 (continued)

Study citation	Sample and characteristics	Reliability evidence	Validity evidence
	Study IV 190 nurses and senior nursing students evaluated written vignettes of TBI patients using LOCFAS	Intrarater: coefficient kappa = .99 for levels; Pearson r = .93 for levels	
Flannery, J. (1995). Cognitive assessment in the acute care setting: Reliability and validity of the Levels of Cognitive Functioning Assessment Scale. *Journal of Nursing Measurement, 3*, 43–58.	Study I 10 doctoral level students in neuropsychology and 2 neuropsychologists assessed videotapes of TBI patients	Interrater: coefficient kappa = 1.00 for levels and .997 for items	
	Study II 177 nurses and nursing students assessed videotapes of TBI patients	Interrater: coefficient kappa = .839 for levels and .830 for items	
	Study III 107 nurses and nursing students assessed videotapes of TBI patients	Intrarater: coefficient kappa = .860 for levels	
	Study IV 5 experts in neuropsychological evaluation and 5 participants from study I assessed videotapes of TBI patients		*Criterion-related validity:* Pearson r = .929 for ratings with LOCFAS and the ranch Los Amigos Levels

TABLE 3.2 (continued)

Study citation	Sample and characteristics	Reliability evidence	Validity evidence
Flannery, J. (1998). Using Levels of Cognitive Functioning Assessment Scale with patients with traumatic brain injury in an acute care setting. *Rehabilitation Nursing*, 23(3), 88–94	28 patients (22 males and 6 females) admitted to one of three acute care facilities. All had sustained traumatic injury to the brain and had admitting diagnoses of closed head injury ($n = 27$) or anoxia ($n = 1$). All were 15 years or older, had a history of normal cognitive functioning and were between Levels I and V on the Rancho at admission.	*Interrater:* Pearson $r = .99$ *Test–Retest:* Pearson $r = .99$[a]	*Criterion-related validity:* Concurrent validity at admission with 4 other instruments, Pearson $r = .85, .86, .89, .91$[b] Concurrent validity with 4 other instruments at discharge, Pearson $r = .86, .90, .94, .94$ Predictive validity between LOCFAS at admission and 4 other instruments at discharge, Pearson $r = .70, .71, .73, .76$

[a]The 4 other instruments were the Glasgow Coma Scale (Teasdale & Jennett, 1974), the Stover-Zeiger Scale (Stover & Zeiger, 1976), the Expanded Glasgow Outcome Scale (Smith, Fields, Lenox, Morris, & Nolan, 1979), and he Disability Rating Scale (Rappaport, Hall, Hopkins, Belleza, and Cope, 1982).

[b]To minimize the confounding of test-retest reliability with recovery, the procedure used by Gouvier, Blanton, LaPorte, and Nepomunceno (1987) was adopted. Each rating was summed across subjects by day of observation. All even numbered observations were then correlated with their preceding odd numbered observations; thus, the resulting Pearson r's reflected the day-to-day stability of the instrument.

CONCLUSIONS AND RECOMMENDATIONS

Results of studies to date indicate that patients who have a low level of responsivity or who are unable to participate appropriately in a comprehensive battery of neuropsychological tests can be assessed reliably and validly using the LOCFAS, which provides a standardized format for communicating about a patient's cognitive functioning. The LOCFAS can also provide nurses with necessary data early in the patient's injury to develop and implement an appropriate plan of care, specific to the patient's strengths and weaknesses, and allow rehabilitation measures to begin much earlier. Through repeated use of the LOCFAS, the patient's progress can be monitored, and ongoing modifications in the care plan can be made to enhance recovery. In addition, appropriate nursing interventions for each of the four levels measured by the LOCFAS have been developed. Table 3.3 shows appropriate nursing interventions for a TBI patient exhibiting Level IV behaviors. (Other levels are available from the author.)

Nurses who care for patients with altered cognitive functioning can be taught to use the LOCFAS as a basis for developing nursing care plans. Appropriate nursing interventions relative to each cognitive level can be established as Standards of Care and included within each patient's plan to enhance early rehabilitation. These nursing interventions are available in the literature (Flannery, 1992, 1997; Hagen et al., 1979; Malkmus, 1983) and are already being implemented in rehabilitation facilities. Undergraduate nursing education can use the LOCFAS to help teach cognitive assessment as a required competency.

In conclusion, although there is clear evidence that supports the reliability and validity of the LOCFAS, data collection should continue and additional reliability and validity assessments will enhance its usefulness. Determination of the impact of training nurses to use the LOCFAS to enhance the reliability and validity of its results is warranted. A study is currently underway to determine the most effective and efficient method for teaching cognitive assessment with the LOCFAS to nurses in acute care settings.

TABLE 3.3 Nursing Management Care Plan for the Patient with Impaired Cognitive Function at Level IV Confused–Agitated

Level IV: Confused–Agitated	

General behaviors:
  Increased agitation
  Patient responding to internal confusion
  Decreased selective attending
  Automatic motor activities present, but internally driven (sits, reaches, ambulates)
Linguistic behaviors
  Overall confusion
  Decreased rate of processing
  Decreased ability to retain, categorize, and associate information
  Decreased attention for graphic processing
  Lack of inhibition to internal stimuli— abusive, or inappropriate language may occur.

Goals	Interventions
Decrease Agitation and Increase Awareness	
Facilitation: Decrease intensity, duration, and frequency of agitation.	Be aware that safety precautions overshadow other measures while the patient is agitated.
Increase attention to the external environment.	If the patient has tubes (feeding, IV, catheters) use mitten splints or elbow restraints to prevent the patient from causing harm to self.
Prevent injury.	If the patient must be left in a regular hospital bed, raise side rails, but pad with pillows or bumpers to prevent the patient from bruising the body.
If possible, have a reliable family member present round-the-clock to soothe and protect the patient from himself, in order not to restrain (this increases agitation exponentially).	
	If no one can stay with the patient, keep a Roll Belt on the patient to prevent him or her from climbing over the side rails or the ends of the bed. Keep bed alarm on. Respond quickly to alarm.
If family cannot stay at the time, see if a sitter (properly trained for Level IV behaviors) can be afforded. If sedating medication can be avoided, the patient will progress more quickly out of this phase.	If one is available in the hospital, transfer the patient to a *Craig bed*, a large padded cubicle with a two mattress-width base resting on the floor. The sides are high enough to prevent the patient from climbing over them. The bottom is wide enough

TABLE 3.3 *(continued)*

Goals	Interventions
Spend adequate time with family to calm them with education about the meaning of the patient's progress through this level	to allow rolling about without any harm. Nurses and other health team members provide care by crawling into the bed with the patient. Freedom from confusing restraints helps prevent added agitation. A net bed may also be used to prevent falling, but eliminates the need for body restraints.
Note: Family members may be terrorized by their loved one's behaviors and believe he/she is worse. It is imperative to help them understand and elicit their help if at all possible. This level can be very brief, depending on many factors.	Continue reorientation x4, introduce yourself and explain all actions, with each encounter.
	Allow "time out" from required measures when agitation is heightened.
	Work on increasing selective attending—specific gross motor tasks, graphic tasks, games, naming of objects.
	Tell the patient "We are working on increasing your attention."
	Modify the environment to decrease external stimuli (lowered lights, lowered noise level, no TV or radio, no unnecessary persons, low voice tones when talking to the patient.
	When the patient's agitation becomes out of control. *DO NOT* try to reason with him or her; he or she cannot process at this time.
	DO: Reduce verbal interaction.
	Attempt to redirect attention. (Distract with a noise or movement; present behavior may be forgotten.)
	Reduce all stimuli; continued discussion will escalate the uncontrolled behavior.

TABLE 3.3 *(continued)*

Goals	Interventions
	Provide physical reassurance—make as comfortable as possible; use gentle or firm touch as needed. If allowed, provide drinks or finger foods. Approach patient indirectly—not head-on—and slowly and quietly.
	Avoid the use of psychotropic drugs because they only have a calming effect when given in large doses, causing decreased cognition. Use medication to calm only as a last resort.
	If the patient is combative, have help available to protect yourself from injury. Learn to stand out of range of casted or splinted limbs; work from weaker side.
	Address inappropriate behavior when it occurs (such as sexual) briefly and simply and go on.

REFERENCES

Brain Injury Association, Inc. (1997). *Fact sheet: traumatic brain injury* [Brochure]. Washington, DC: Author.

Brooks, N. (1984). Cognitive deficits after head injury. In N. Brooks (Ed.), *Closed head injury: Psychological, social and family consequences* (pp. 43–73). New York: Oxford University Press.

Craine, S. (1982). Principles of cognitive rehabilitation. In L. Trexler (Ed.). *Cognitive rehabilitation: Conceptualization and intervention* (pp. 83–97). New York: Plenum.

Eames, P., & Wood, R. (1985). Rehabilitation after severe brain injury: A follow-up study of the behavior modification approach. *Journal of Neurology, Neurosurgery, and Psychiatry, 48,* 613–610.

Flannery, J. (1987). Validity and reliability of the Levels of Cognitive Functioning Assessment Scale for adults with closed head injuries. (Doctoral dissertation, University of Alabama at Birmingham, 1987). *Dissertation Abstracts International, 48,* 32488.

Flannery, J. (1992). Nursing management of adults with common problems of the nervous system. In L. O. Burrell (Ed), *Adult nursing in hospital and community settings* (pp. 864–924). Norwalk, CT: Appleton-Lange.

Flannery, J. (1993). Psychometric properties of a cognitive functioning scale for TBI patients. *Western Journal of Nursing Research, 15*(4), 465–482.

Flannery, J. (1995). Cognitive assessment in the acute care setting: Reliability of the Levels of Cognitive Functioning Assessment Scale. *Journal of Nursing Measurement, 3*, 43–58.

Flannery, J. (1997). Common neurological interventions. In L. O. Burrell, M. Gerlach, & B. Pless (Eds.), *Adult nursing: Acute and community care* (pp. 880–926). Norwalk, CT: Appleton & Lange.

Flannery, J. (1998). Using the Levels of Cognitive Functioning Assessment Scale with patients with traumatic brain injury in an acute care setting. *Rehabilitation Nursing, 23*(3), 88–94.

Gouvier, W., Blanton, P., LaPorte K., & Nepomuceno, C. (1987). Reliability and validity of the Disability Rating Scale and the Levels of Cognitive Functioning Scale in monitoring recovery from severe head injury. *Archives of Physical Medicine and Rehabilitation, 68*, 94–97.

Hagen, C. (1982). Language—cognitive disorganization following closed head injury. A conceptualization. In L. Trexler (Ed.), Cognitive *rehabilitation: Conceptualization and intervention* (pp. 143–151). New York: Plenum.

Hagen, C., Malkmus, D., & Durham, P. (1979). Levels of cognitive functioning. In *Rehabilitation of the head injured adult: Comprehensive physical management* (pp. 87–89). Downey, CA: Professional Staff Associates of Rancho Los Amigos Hospital.

Levin, J. S., Benton, A., & Grossman, R. (1982). *Neurobehavioral consequences of closed head injury.* New York: Oxford University Press.

Luria, A. (1973). *The working brain.* New York: Basic Books.

Malkmus, D. (1983). Integrating cognitive strategies into the physical therapy setting. *Physical Therapy, 63*(12), 1952–1959.

Malkmus, D., Booth, B., & Kodimer, C. (1980). *Rehabilitation of the head-injured adult: Comprehensive cognitive management.* Downey, CA: Professional Staff Association of Rancho Los Amigos Hospital.

Neuman, B. (1995). *The Neuman Systems Model* (3rd ed.) Stamford, CT: Appleton, & Lange.

Stover, S., & Zeiger, N. (1976). Head injury in children and teenagers: Functional recovery correlated with duration of coma. *Archives of Physical Medicine and Rehabilitation, 57*, 201–205.

Warren, J., & Peck, J. (1984). Factors which influence neuropsychological recovery from severe head injury. *Journal of Neurosurgical Nursing, 16*, 248–251.

APPENDIX: DIRECTIONS TO EXAMINER USING LEVELS OF COGNITIVE FUNCTIONING ASSESSMENT SCALE

1. Stamp record with Addressograph or write patient's name and birth date.
2. Enter diagnosis and date of injury and onset of cognitive deficits.
3. Record the date and time of examination and your initials at the top of the column to be used.
4. Record your legal signature with your initials on the back page of the record.
5. After familiarizing yourself with the clustered behaviors in each level described on LOCFAS, begin to observe the patient without disturbing him/her for a few minutes (3–5). From this brief observation of his/her random interaction with uncontrolled environmental stimuli, you will have a general idea of what level to anticipate (Level I as opposed to Level V).
6. Proceed to observe and elicit responses and mark the box beside the observed behavior in the appropriate column. A single column is used for each assessment. Continue upward on the scale assessing for observable behaviors for each level. Cease assessment at the point that no expected behaviors for a whole level can be observed. The cognitive level is designated as the *highest* level at which the *preponderance* of matching behavioral responses occur. There is always a scatter of responses above and below this level. The next higher level in which two or more behaviors are checked is also recorded. The patient is assessed for his best effort since these behaviors indicate the patient's capacity to move up to a higher level. There is expected a certain amount of overlap between levels, since human behavior is not precise. Variation downward during the day, particularly in relation to distractions, fatigue, and stress, is expected to occur.
7. As the patient progresses up the Levels, the team may want to give three separate scores—cognitive, behavioral, and functional—since there can be such variations among these areas. For example, the patient may clearly respond cognitively to stimuli on a Level V and physically is able to execute most tasks, but behaviorally he chooses not to do them (without expressing these thoughts). A quick assessment without follow-up would lead the observers to believe the patient is on a lower cognitive level.
8. The assessment may take approximately fifteen minutes. It can be incorporated within other aspects of routine care and therefore no exact time frame is set. Observations begin with the caregiver's first encounter with the patient and may extend through whatever activities in which the patient and caregiver normally engage until adequate assessment data are gathered.

9. The LOCFAS has a grid that accommodates an ongoing assessment over time. The frequency of recording is relative to the stability of the patient's condition and the number of team members assessing the patient. It is appropriate for use by an interdisciplinary health team. Accumulated data from all sources over time provide an accurate assessment, generally discussed by the team on a weekly basis. Progression, or regression, if any, can readily be determined from the overall evaluation.

10. Absence of the opportunity to observe these behaviors does not affect the decision regarding the cognitive level. In certain situations the precipitating stimulus may be absent. For example in Level II, Behavior 10, referring to change in level of activity upon repeated stimuli, may not be observed because it was not possible to provide stimuli repetitively. However, if more behaviors were observed in Level II than in any other level, the patient would still be ranked Level II without Behavior 10.

LEVELS OF COGNITIVE FUNCTIONING ASSESSMENT SCALE

Developed by Jeanne Flannery using Levels 1–5 from Rancho Los Amigos Scale

Date ☐ ☐ ☐ ☐ ☐ ☐
Time ☐ ☐ ☐ ☐ ☐ ☐
Initials ☐ ☐ ☐ ☐ ☐ ☐

Level I. <u>NO RESPONSE</u>

A. Attention to the Environment: NONE
   1. Appears unaware of environment; eyes usually closed   1. ☐ ☐ ☐ ☐ ☐ ☐
B. Response to Stimuli: NONE
   2. Completely unresponsive to tactile stimuli and position changes   2. ☐ ☐ ☐ ☐ ☐ ☐
   3. Completely unresponsive to auditory stimuli   3. ☐ ☐ ☐ ☐ ☐ ☐
   4. Completely unresponsive to visual stimuli (This is not to be confused with papillary response to light, which is reflexive.)   4. ☐ ☐ ☐ ☐ ☐ ☐
   5. Completely unresponsive to painful stimuli   5. ☐ ☐ ☐ ☐ ☐ ☐
   6. Completely unresponsive to gustatory stimuli   6. ☐ ☐ ☐ ☐ ☐ ☐
C. Behavior Status: REFLEXIVE
   7. May have primitive responses such as snorting, chewing, blinking, eye opening, which are unrelated to specific stimuli   7. ☐ ☐ ☐ ☐ ☐ ☐
D. Ability to Process Information: NONE
E. Ability to Follow Commands: NONE
F. Awareness of Person (Self):   NONE

G. Awareness of Time: NONE
H. Ability to Perform Self-Care: NONE
I. Ability to Converse: NONE
J. Ability to Learn New Information: NONE

Date ☐ ☐ ☐ ☐ ☐ ☐
Time ☐ ☐ ☐ ☐ ☐ ☐
Initials ☐ ☐ ☐ ☐ ☐ ☐

Level II. <u>GENERALIZED RESPONSE</u>

A. Attention to Environment: NONE
B. Response to Stimuli: NONSPECIFIC, INCONSISTENT

   8. May respond to external stimuli, such as position changes, with physiologic changes such as increased BP, P, or R, or increased perspiration   8. ☐ ☐ ☐ ☐ ☐ ☐

   9. Responds to painful stimuli with generalized reflex action (nonpurposeful gross body movement, as decerebration or decortication)   9. ☐ ☐ ☐ ☐ ☐ ☐

  10. Repetitive stimuli produce a change in the level of response, either dampening or heightening it (e.g. stroking may reduce physiologic changes or intensify response, which occurred initially)   10. ☐ ☐ ☐ ☐ ☐ ☐

  11. Demonstrates nonpurposeful variations in responses to the same stimulus; delayed, limited response   11. ☐ ☐ ☐ ☐ ☐ ☐

C. Behavior Status: AWAKE

  12. May be awake but unaware of environment unless directly stimulated   12. ☐ ☐ ☐ ☐ ☐ ☐

  13. Demonstrates inconsistent infrequent visual fixation; may have roving eye movements, but is incapable of visual tracking   13. ☐ ☐ ☐ ☐ ☐ ☐

  14. Behavioral response may be the same regardless of stimulus (e.g. eye opening, startle, gross body movement, or decerebration upon tactile, painful, or auditory stimulus)   14. ☐ ☐ ☐ ☐ ☐ ☐

D. Ability to Process Information: NONE
E. Ability to Follow Commands: NONE
F. Awareness of Person (Self): STIMULI TO BODY PRODUCE GENERAL RESPONSE
G. Awareness of Time (Present): NONE
H. Ability to Perform Self-Care: NONE
I. Ability to Converse: NONE
J. Ability to Learn New Information: NONE

Date ☐ ☐ ☐ ☐ ☐ ☐
Time ☐ ☐ ☐ ☐ ☐ ☐
Initials ☐ ☐ ☐ ☐ ☐ ☐

Level III. <u>LOCALIZED RESPONSE</u>

A. Attention to the Environment: NONE
B. Response to Stimuli: SPECIFIC,
                                                          INCONSISTENT
   15. Tracks briefly a moving object in visual field   15. ☐ ☐ ☐ ☐ ☐ ☐
      when awake only if stimulus intensity gains
      attention; inconsistent response
   16. Demonstrates withdrawal responses or facial   16. ☐ ☐ ☐ ☐ ☐ ☐
      grimacing to tactile stimuli (pressure,
      temperature, texture) but inconsistently
   17. Responds specifically to the stimulus (e.g.   17. ☐ ☐ ☐ ☐ ☐ ☐
      resists restraints, swallows food, relaxes
      to stroking, pulls at NGT) but inconsistently
   18. Responds inconsistently to same stimulus   18. ☐ ☐ ☐ ☐ ☐ ☐
      (e.g. turns toward or away from a sound)
C. Behavior Status: BEGINNING AWARENESS
   19. Awakens to stimuli; has sleep/wake cycles;   19. ☐ ☐ ☐ ☐ ☐ ☐
      awakens spontaneously
   20. Demonstrates purposeful visual orientation   20. ☐ ☐ ☐ ☐ ☐ ☐
      and fixation
   21. Moves body parts purposefully, if able   21. ☐ ☐ ☐ ☐ ☐ ☐
D. Ability to Process Information: NONE
E. Ability to Follow Commands: INCONSISTENT,
                                                            DELAYED
   22. Response to commands is delayed   22. ☐ ☐ ☐ ☐ ☐ ☐
   23. Responds more consistently with some persons   23. ☐ ☐ ☐ ☐ ☐ ☐
      than with others (e.g. may look at regular care-
      giver when called, but may not do it with others)
   24. Demonstrates inconsistent attention   24. ☐ ☐ ☐ ☐ ☐ ☐
      and language comprehension, but when there
      is a response it is unequivocally meaningful
      (e.g. may not respond to command "touch
      your nose" when it has been followed before)
F. Awareness of Person (Self):   VAGUE, NOT
                                                          MEASURABLE
G. Awareness of Time (Present):   VAGUE, NOT
                                                          MEASURABLE
H. Ability to Perform Self-Care: NONE
I. Ability to Converse: INCONSISTENT
   25. May vocalize inconsistently to stimuli; but   25. ☐ ☐ ☐ ☐ ☐ ☐
      may be infrequent
   26. May vocalize automatically with one or   26. ☐ ☐ ☐ ☐ ☐ ☐
      two-word response or just make loud noises
J. Ability to Learn New Information: NONE

Date ☐ ☐ ☐ ☐ ☐ ☐
Time ☐ ☐ ☐ ☐ ☐ ☐
Initials ☐ ☐ ☐ ☐ ☐ ☐

Level IV. CONFUSED—AGITATED

A. Attention to the Environment: BRIEF
   27. Demonstrates fleeting general attention to   27. ☐ ☐ ☐ ☐ ☐ ☐
       surroundings; unable to concentrate
   28. Selective attention may be nonexistent or so   28. ☐ ☐ ☐ ☐ ☐ ☐
       brief that is not acted upon; easily distractible
B. Response to Stimuli: SPECIFIC, INAPPROPRIATE
   29. May respond consistently to a stimulus, but the   29. ☐ ☐ ☐ ☐ ☐ ☐
       response is inappropriate because of internal
       confusion
   30. May become very agitated or yell in response to   30. ☐ ☐ ☐ ☐ ☐ ☐
       a mild stimulus and sustain response after
       stimulus removed; "sticks" in response; low
       tolerance for frustration or pain
   31. Responds to presence of devices, attachments or   31. ☐ ☐ ☐ ☐ ☐ ☐
       anything confining with strong, persistent,
       purposeful attempt to remove; impatient; demanding
C. Behavior Status: AGITATED, CONFUSED
   32. In a heightened state of activity related to internal   32. ☐ ☐ ☐ ☐ ☐ ☐
       agitation (environment may be quiet and
       nonstimulating); restless; pacing; rocking,
       rubbing; moaning
   33. May demonstrate aggressive, hostile behavior; has   33. ☐ ☐ ☐ ☐ ☐ ☐
       explosive or unpredictable anger; may be self
       abusive
   34. May show sudden changes in mood (e.g. crying,   34. ☐ ☐ ☐ ☐ ☐ ☐
       laughter, anger, or sleep)
   35. Performs overlearned motor activities automatically,   35. ☐ ☐ ☐ ☐ ☐ ☐
       but may resist commands to do these same
       activities, such as "sit up"
D. Ability to Process Information: MINIMAL
   36. Unable to understand or cooperate with treatment   36. ☐ ☐ ☐ ☐ ☐ ☐
       efforts; may be combative; resistant to care;
       will leave area, if able
E. Ability to Follow Commands: INCONSISTENT
   37. May respond briefly or inconsistently to simple   37. ☐ ☐ ☐ ☐ ☐ ☐
       commands when agitation is lessened
F. Awareness of Person (Self):   ORIENTED X1
   38. Is oriented to own name; aware of own body   38. ☐ ☐ ☐ ☐ ☐ ☐
G. Awareness of Time (Present):   NONE
   39. Unaware of present events; responds primarily   39. ☐ ☐ ☐ ☐ ☐ ☐
       to own state of severe confusion
H. Ability to Perform Self-Care: MINIMAL
   40. Performs self care activities for brief periods with   40. ☐ ☐ ☐ ☐ ☐ ☐
       maximum direction and cuing; cannot focus
       without redirection

I. Ability to Converse: PRESENT, INAPPROPRIATE
    41. Verbalizes incoherently or with words unrelated to 41.☐ ☐ ☐ ☐ ☐ ☐
        the current situation; talking may be rapid, loud,
        excessive
    42. May confabulate (give incorrect answers to 42.☐ ☐ ☐ ☐ ☐ ☐
        questions about the present from unrelated
        long-term memory stores); lacks short-term recall
    43. Conversation reflects confusion and memory deficits 43.☐ ☐ ☐ ☐ ☐ ☐
J. Ability to Learn New Information: NONE

                            Date ☐ ☐ ☐ ☐ ☐ ☐
                            Time ☐ ☐ ☐ ☐ ☐ ☐
                       Initials ☐ ☐ ☐ ☐ ☐ ☐

Level V. <u>CONFUSED—INAPPROPRIATE, NON AGITATED</u>

A. Attention to Environment: DISTRACTIBLE
    44. Demonstrates gross attention consistently 44.☐ ☐ ☐ ☐ ☐ ☐
    45. Has difficulty sustaining selective attention; highly 45.☐ ☐ ☐ ☐ ☐ ☐
        distractible; limited concentration
    46. Lacks ability to focus on a specific thing without 46.☐ ☐ ☐ ☐ ☐ ☐
        frequent redirection
B. Response to Stimuli: VARIABLE
    47. Responds readily to stimuli related to self, body 47.☐ ☐ ☐ ☐ ☐ ☐
        comfort, family
    48. Use of objects in environment often inappropriate, 48.☐ ☐ ☐ ☐ ☐ ☐
        without direction
C. Behavior Status: INAPPROPRIATE
    49. Unable to initiate functional tasks 49.☐ ☐ ☐ ☐ ☐ ☐
    50. May demonstrate frustration and negative, 50.☐ ☐ ☐ ☐ ☐ ☐
        inappropriate behaviors in response to external
        stimuli, usually out of proportion to stimulus
    51. Will tend to wander (on foot or in a wheel chair) 51.☐ ☐ ☐ ☐ ☐ ☐
        from unit; will not remember a command to
        remain in a certain place; will not remember how
        to return from a strange area to a familiar place
D. Ability to Process Information: LIMITED TO SELF
    52. May relate to conversation about own body 52.☐ ☐ ☐ ☐ ☐ ☐
        comfort, personal needs, momentary concerns
E. Ability to Follow Commands: CONSISTENT, IF
                         SIMPLE
    53. Responds to single simple commands consistently 53.☐ ☐ ☐ ☐ ☐ ☐
    54. Response to a complex command becomes 54.☐ ☐ ☐ ☐ ☐ ☐
        fragmented, nonpurposeful, and unrelated to
        command; requires redirection to follow through
F. Awareness of Person (Self):   ORIENTED X1
    55. Oriented to self; knows name, special things 55.☐ ☐ ☐ ☐ ☐ ☐
        about self, but not how the present self is
        different from past
G. Awareness of Time (Present):   CONFUSED
    56. Disoriented to time and place, confusing past 56.☐ ☐ ☐ ☐ ☐ ☐
        and present; unaware of situation

57. Demonstrates severe short-term memory deficit 57. ☐ ☐ ☐ ☐ ☐ ☐

H. Ability to Perform Self-Care: REQUIRES
                                   MAXIMUM
                                   ASSISTANCE

58. Performs overlearned tasks with maximum structure 58. ☐ ☐ ☐ ☐ ☐ ☐
and cuing, but does not initiate the activity

I. Ability to Converse: SOCIAL-AUTOMATIC

59. May converse on a social-automatic level for 59. ☐ ☐ ☐ ☐ ☐ ☐
short periods, as "I'm fine, how are you?", but
responses are often unrelated to specific topics
of conversation

60. If not verbal, may use social-automatic gestures, 60. ☐ ☐ ☐ ☐ ☐ ☐
as shoulder shrug, thumbs, up

J. Ability to Learn New Information: NONE

61. Unable to learn new tasks; even though tries, 61. ☐ ☐ ☐ ☐ ☐ ☐
listens, follows commands, outcome not achieved.

Date ☐ ☐ ☐ ☐ ☐ ☐
Time ☐ ☐ ☐ ☐ ☐ ☐
Initials ☐ ☐ ☐ ☐ ☐ ☐

SUMMARY

62. Select a number from 1 to 5 which represents the 62. ☐ ☐ ☐ ☐ ☐ ☐
highest Cognitive Level where *most* of the
observed behaviors are checked at this time
of observation

Signature	Title	Initials	Signature	Title	Initials

4

Evaluating Older Persons for Cognitive Impairment: The Abilities Assessment Instrument

Donna L. Wells, Pam Dawson, Souraya Sidani, and Jennifer Cutler

This chapter discusses the Abilities Assessment Instrument (AAI), which evaluates elders for cognitive impairment.

PURPOSE

The Abilities Assessment Instrument (AAI) was developed by Dawson, Wells, Reid, and Sidani (1998) to evaluate elders for cognitive impairment. It was designed to help caregivers ascertain the extent to which abilities are retained in four areas: self-care, social, interactional, and interpretive abilities. The AAI was based on a description of the abilities that underlie certain activities and suggests particular nursing interventions that may promote retained abilities and compensate for those that have been lost (Dawson, Wells, & Kline, 1993; Wells & Dawson, 2000). Therefore, it is unique because it links the behaviors observed in clinical practice to the clinical features of dementia in order to understand those abilities affected by the disease and how daily functioning is consequently affected. The AAI provides the nurse with an instrument that can be used to guide the assessment and selection of specific nursing interventions that are appropriate to the elder's ability level.

CONCEPTUAL BASIS OF THE ABILITIES ASSESSMENT
INSTRUMENT

Delineation of the conceptual basis of the AAI involved a careful review of the literature to identify indicators of abilities in older persons. The research literature about dementia was critically analyzed to determine the abilities that people potentially retain. Categorization of the four ability areas on the AAI are congruent with the cardinal features of dementia, which have been organized as problems with movement and praxis, attention, language, and memory and depression (Hart & Semple, 1990). The categories of retained abilities also reflect those that are important for daily living and that can be addressed by nursing care.

Specifically, the self-care abilities noted from the review included voluntary movements, spatial orientation, initiation and follow-through, and purposeful movements. The ability of voluntary movements incorporates the particular abilities related to movement of lips, fingers, and arms, which may be affected with dementia by the presence of the suck and grasp reflexes and paratonia (Bakchine, Lacomblez, Palisson, Laurent, & Derouesne, 1989; Vreeling, Houx, Jolles, & Verhey, 1995). Spatial orientation is reflected by the abilities of left/right orientation and finding one's way, which are challenged by spatial disorientation (DeLeon, Potegal, & Gurland, 1984; Liu, Gauthier, & Gauthier, 1991). Initiation and follow-through and purposeful movements may be affected by the apraxias (Rapcsak, Croswell, & Rubens, 1989; Taylor, 1994) and perseveration (Bayles, Tomoeda, & Kaszniak, 1985), which are demonstrated by the specific abilities of performing activities in relation to object use.

The area of social abilities consists of those abilities concerned with giving and receiving attention, as well as engaging in conversation. The threatened ability of attention incorporates social greeting, humor, and music abilities, which are affected by attentional dysfunction (Adasiak, 1989; Capitani, Della Sala, Lucchelli, Soave, & Spinnler, 1988). Staying on topic, verbal response, and nonverbal response are the particular items that reflect the ability of conversation, which may be affected by the impaired use of the rules of language (Hutchinson & Jensen, 1980; Kempler, 1988).

The capacities to comprehend and express language are involved in the area of interactional abilities. Language comprehension incorporates the specific abilities to understand verbal and written commands and yes/no sentences. These abilities are affected by aphasia (Cummings, Benson, Hill, & Read, 1985). Language expression involves verbal and written object identification and sentence completion. Both are affected by anomia and aphasia (Bayles & Tomoeda, 1983; Huff, Corkin, & Growden, 1986; Martin & Fedio, 1983).

The area of interpretive abilities is composed of those related to recognition, including the abilities of (1) self-, facial affect-, object-, and time-recognition; (2) recall of familiar objects and places; and (3) subjective feeling states. These specific abilities are affected by memory impairment (Albert, Cohen, & Koff, 1991; Carlesimo, Sabbadini, Fadda, & Caltagirone, 1995; Diesfeldt, 1990; Fromholt & Larsen, 1991; Grewal, 1994; Migliorelli et al., 1995; Randolph, Tierney, & Chase, 1995; Sainsbury & Coristine, 1986) and depression (Burt, Zembar, & Niederehe, 1995).

PROCEDURES FOR DEVELOPMENT

The original instrument consisted of 58 items generated to measure the specific abilities organized into the self-care, social, interactional, and interpretive categories. Assessment methods were devised to measure the retention of each of the specific abilities and were guided by the literature. Appropriateness of the items and related assessments was determined by conducting a pilot study in which 100 evaluations were made of individuals with dementia who lived in the community or an institution. The purpose of the pilot study was to determine if each item was appropriate, if it accurately assessed for the ability of interest, and if the assessment finding was useful in selecting a nursing intervention. Results of the pilot study indicated that persons with dementia were able to participate in the assessment and that nurses were able to identify these persons' potentially retained abilities. The final version of the AAI (before testing) included 58 items, divided into four subscales reflecting the self-care (12 items), social (10 items), interactional (18 items), and interpretive (18 items) abilities.

Five experts in the care of older persons assessed content validity. Two of them were clinical nurse specialists, two were faculty members in gerontological nursing, and one was a geriatric psychiatrist. These experts were provided with a written description of the instrument, the instrument itself, and a Content Validity Questionnaire developed by the investigators following the content validity assessment procedure Lynn (1986) described. They independently rated the degree to which the instrument's format and its content, in terms of its 12 categories and 58 items, reflected what the instrument was designed to measure on a scale that ranged from 3 (agree) to 1 (disagree). More specifically, each of the categories and items was rated on clarity and representativeness. The index of content validity (CVI) reflected the percent agreement of the judges across the items (Waltz, Strickland, & Lenz, 1991).

A CVI of 87.3% was obtained, indicating that at least four of the five judges were in agreement that the subscales and the majority of items measured the abilities of elderly persons with cognitive impairment. For eight of the 58 items, there was less than 80% agreement. Two of the five judges questioned the representativeness of the items in measuring a particular ability and/or the clarity of the item's wording.

The internal consistency reliability of the AAI was examined, using the data collected in the pilot study. Analysis of the item-to-total correlation was done for each of the four subscales. Results indicated that some items in the social, interactional, and interpretive subscales had a low (< .30) item-to-total subscale correlation. Therefore, these items were deleted from their respective subscales, and the Cronbach's alpha coefficients were reestimated for the three subscales. The coefficients were .92 for the social (9 items), .99 for the interactional (17 items), and .98 for the interpretive subscales (18 items).

DESCRIPTION

Each of the four areas of abilities is assessed/measured with a subscale. The number of items in each subscale varies. The total number of items was 58 before testing and 55 following the psychometric evaluation. (See Appendix for updated instrument.)

Administration and Scoring

The AAI is an assessment tool that is designed to be administered by clinicians. Clinicians are trained in eliciting the behavior(s) inquired about in each item, observing the patients' responses, and selecting the appropriate response option to record their observations. Most of the items are scored dichotomously to indicate retained or lost abilities. The remaining items are scored continuously to capture the degree of the ability retained. The potential range of scores is 0 to 186 for the total instrument, 0 to 44 for self-care abilities, 0 to 29 for social abilities, 0 to 66 for interactional abilities, and 0 to 44 for interpretive abilities. The higher the score on the items, the greater the retained ability.

RELIABILITY AND VALIDITY EVIDENCE

Initial Assessment of the AAI

The initial psychometric evaluation of the AAI was conducted on a sample of male veterans. The veterans received care in a 670–bed extended-care department of a university hospital in metropolitan Toronto. The AAI was found to be a reliable and valid instrument that can be used to assess the abilities of older people with dementia (Dawson et al., 1998). The psychometric evaluation of the AAI indicated that it is reliable (1) in terms of test–retest (Pearson's *r* range .93 to .99), interrater (Pearson's *r* range .95 to .99), and internal consistency evaluations (Cronbach's alpha

= .90 to .98), as well as (2) through confirmatory factor analysis. It is valid with respect to: (1) content validity (CVI 87.3%), (2) concurrent validity (Pearson's *r* correlations ranging from –.67 to .80 on the London Psychogeriatric Rating Scale [LPRS; Hersch, Kral, & Palmer, 1978], and from –.76 to .85 on the Functional Assessment Stages Scale [FAST; Reisberg, Ferris, & Franssen, 1985], and (3) construct validity, with significant differences between subjects with or without cognitive impairment (*t* values ranging from 5.13 to 9.30). Based on the assessment results, which indicate abilities retained or lost, caregivers would be able to design appropriate caregiving approaches that promote retained abilities or compensate for lost ones.

Subsequent Testing of the AAI

Two Master of Science nursing students conducted psychometric studies of the social and self-care components of the AAI on different samples. Their findings offered further confirmation of Dawson and colleagues' (1998) results (Lyle & Wells, 1997; Rivera, 1998). Rivera's research on the reliability and validity of the AAI's social abilities component in a population of elderly women (30 with cognitive impairment and 30 without), demonstrated: (1) test–retest reliability (r = .95, $p < .001$); (2) interrater reliability (100%); (3) internal consistency (Cronbach's alpha = .66); (4) content validity (CVI = .95); (5) construct validity ($t = -8.2$, $p = .001$); and (6) concurrent validity (r = .74, $p < .001$). Lyle and Wells's study of the reliability and validity of the AAI's self-care component for elderly women residing in long-term care who had cognitive impairment ($n = 30$), or for those participating in an associated day-care program who had no evidence of cognitive impairment ($n = 20$) indicated: (1) test–retest reliability (r_s = .79, $p < .01$, $n = 10$); (2) interrater agreement (r_s = .97, $p < .01$, n = 9]; (3) internal consistency (Cronbach's alpha = .97); (4) content validity (CVI = .89); (5) concurrent validity (r_s = .91, $p < .01$); and (6) construct validity (Mann-Whitney $U = 85$). The Mini-Mental State Examination (Folstein, Folstein, & McHugh, 1975) was used to determine concurrent validity in both studies.

CONCLUSIONS AND RECOMMENDATIONS

Further psychometric testing of the AAI is needed with larger and more diverse samples of older persons with dementia. Researchers beginning work in this area have reported reliability and validity: (1) for the AAI's self-care subscale in a sample of women residing either in a long-term care facility or in the community (Lyle & Wells, 1997); (2) for the AAI's social abilities subscale in a sample of women in an acute care setting

(Rivera, 1998), and (3) for the AAI in a population of male veterans (Dawson et al., 1998). To test and expand this descriptive theory of retained abilities and to account for the limitations of these studies, which include single sites and homogeneous populations, future investigators might explore and compare the nature of retained abilities in other populations, for example, female and male persons with dementia who reside at home or in other types of long-term care facilities. Cross-cultural responses on the AAI could also be investigated. Further investigation could test: (1) how the results of the assessment can guide the selection of interventions, (2) the clinical utility of the AAI, and (3) its use to assess the effectiveness of selected interventions, such as sensitivity to change.

The findings from testing the AAI offer support for a positive approach to caregiving that emphasizes abilities. Enhancing the abilities of people, such as those who are suffering from dementia, requires a knowledge of remaining or retained abilities. Regardless of the degree to which abilities are retained, the caregiving objective is to promote and to compensate for (i.e. assist with caregiving) only those abilities that are noted to be preserved at a moderate or low level. The implication for practice concerning people with dementia is that individualized assessments and care plans that detail their level and type of abilities can, and should, be developed. In order to develop an effective, individualized plan of care, caregivers must be able to assess abilities based on an objective measurement of observed behavior. The AAI provides nurses with a reliable and valid instrument that can be used to select specific nursing interventions to help persons who suffer from dementia. These interventions can be based on sound knowledge of patients' strengths and weaknesses.

REFERENCES

Adasiak, J. P. (1989). Humor and the Alzheimer's patient: The psychological basis. *The American Journal of Alzheimer's Care and Related Disorders & Research, 4*(4), 18–21.

Albert, M. S., Cohen, C., & Koff, E. (1991). Perception of affect in patients with dementia of the Alzheimer type. *Archives of Neurology, 48*, 791–795.

Bakchine, S., Lacomblez, L., Palisson, E., Laurent, M., & Derouesne, C. (1989). Relationship between primitive reflexes, extra-pyramidal signs, reflective apraxia and severity of cognitive impairment in dementia of the Alzheimer type. *Acta Neurologica Scandinavica, 79*, 38–46.

Bayles, K., & Tomoeda, C. (1983). Confrontation naming impairment in dementia. *Brain and Language, 19*, 98–114.

Bayles, K. A., Tomoeda, C. K., & Kaszniak, A. W. (1985). Verbal perseveration of dementia patients. *Brain and Language, 25*, 102–116.

Burt, D. B., Zembar, J. J., & Niederehe, G. (1995). Depression and memory impairment: A meta-analysis of the association, its pattern, and specificity. *Psychological Bulletin, 117*, 285–305.

Capitani, E., Della Sala, S., Lucchelli, F., Soave, P., & Spinnler, H. (1988). Gottschaldt's hidden figure test: Sensitivity of perceptual attention to ageing and dementia. *Journal of Gerontology, 43*, 157–163.

Carlesimo, G. A., Sabbadini, M., Fadda, L., & Caltagirone, C. (1995). Forgetting from long-term memory in dementia and pure amnesia: Role of task, delay of assessment and aetiology of cerebral damage. *Cortex, 31*, 285–300.

Cummings, J., Benson, F., Hill, M., & Read, S. (1985). Aphasia in dementia of the Alzheimer type. *Neurology, 35*, 394–397.

Dawson, P., Wells, D., & Kline, K. (1993). *Enhancing the abilities of persons with Alzheimer's and related dementias: A nursing perspective.* New York: Springer Publishing Co.

Dawson, P., Wells, D. L., Reid, D., & Sidani, S. (1998). An abilities assessment instrument for elderly persons with cognitive impairment: Psychometric properties and clinical utility. *Journal of Nursing Measurement, 6*(1), 35–54.

DeLeon, M. J., Potegal, M., & Gurland, B. (1984). Wandering and parietal signs in senile dementia of the Alzheimer's type. *Neuropsychobiology, 11*, 155–157.

Diesfeldt, H. F. A. (1990). Recognition memory for words and faces in primary degenerative dementia of the Alzheimer type and normal old age *Journal of Clinical and Experimental Neuropsychology, 12*, 931–945.

Folstein, M. F., Folstein, S., & McHugh, P. R. (1975). Mini-Mental State: A practical method for grading the cognitive state of patients for the clinician. *Journal of Psychiatric Research, 12*, 189–198.

Fromholt, P., & Larsen, S. F. (1991). Autobiographical memory in normal aging and primary degenerative dementia (dementia of the Alzheimer type). *Journal of Psychiatric Research, 12*, 85–91.

Grewal, R. P. (1994). Self-recognition in dementia of the Alzheimer type. *Perceptual & Motor Skills, 79*(2), 1009–1010.

Hart S., & Semple, J. M. (1990). *Neuropsychology and the dementias.* London: Taylor & Francis.

Hersch, E. L., Kral, V. A., & Palmer, R. B. (1978). Clinical value of the London Psychogeriatric Rating Scale. *Journal of the American Geriatrics Society, 26*, 348–354.

Huff, J., Corkin, S., & Growden, J. (1986). Semantic impairment and anomia in Alzheimer's disease. *Brain and Language, 28*, 235–249.

Hutchinson J. M., & Jensen, M. (1980). A pragmatic evaluation of discourse communication in normal and senile elderly in a nursing home. In L. Obler & M. Albert (Eds.), *Language and communication in the elderly* (pp.   ). Lexington, Massachusetts: Lexington Books.

Kempler, D. (1988). Lexical and pantomime abilities in Alzheimer's disease. *Aphasiology, 2*, 343–350.

Liu, L., Gauthier, L. L., & Gauthier, S. (1991). Spatial disorientation in persons with early senile dementia of the Alzheimer type. *The American Journal of Occupational Therapy, 45*(1), 67–74.

Lyle C. M., & Wells, D. L. (1997). Description of a self-care instrument for elders. *Western Journal of Nursing Research, 19,* 637–653.

Lynn, M. R. (1986). Determination and quantification of content validity. *Nursing Research, 35,* 382–385.

Martin A., & Fedio, P. (1983). Word production and comprehension in Alzheimer's disease: The breakdown of semantic knowledge. *Brain and Language, 19,* 124–141.

Migliorelli, R., Teson, A., Sabe, L., Petracca, G., Petracchi, M., Leiguarda, R., & Starkstein, S. E. (1995). Anosognosia in Alzheimer's disease: A study of associated factors. *Journal of Neuropsychiatry & Clinical Neurosciences, 7,* 338–344.

Randolph, C., Tierney, M. C., & Chase, T. N. (1995). Implicit memory in Alzheimer's disease. *Journal of Clinical & Experimental Neuropsychology, 17,* 343–351.

Rapcsak, S. Z., Croswell, S. C., & Rubens, A. B. (1989). Apraxia in Alzheimer's disease. *Neurology, 39,* 664–668.

Reisberg, B., Ferris, S. H., & Franssen, E. (1985). An ordinal functional assessment tool for Alzheimer's-type dementia. *Hospital and Community Psychiatry, 36,* 593–595.

Rivera, T. (1998). Reliability and validity of the social abilities component of an abilities assessment instrument. *Perspectives, 22*(3), 16–26.

Sainsbury R. S., & Coristine, M. (1986). Affective discrimination in moderately to severely demented patients. *Canadian Journal on Aging, 5,* 99–104.

Taylor, R. (1994). Motor apraxia in dementia. *Perceptual and Motor Skills, 79,* 523–528.

Vreeling, F. W., Houx, P. J., Jolles, J., & Verhey, F. R. (1995). Primitive reflexes in Alzheimer's disease and vascular dementia. *Journal of Geriatric Psychiatry & Neurology, 8*(2), 111–117.

Waltz, C. F., Strickland, O. L., & Lenz, E. R. (1991). *Measurement in nursing research* (2nd ed.). Philadelphia: F. A. Davis.

Wells, D. L., & Dawson, P. (2000). Description of retained abilities in older persons with dementia. *Research in Nursing & Health, 23,* 158–166.

APPENDIX: ABILITIES ASSESSMENT FOR THE NURSING CARE OF PERSONS WITH ALZHEIMER'S DISEASE AND RELATED DISORDERS*

Name:

Age:

Visual Impairment   Yes ____ No ____

Hearing Impairment: Yes ____ No ____

Medical Diagnosis:

SCORE:				
	Self-Care Abilities	____(39)	Percentage	____(100)
	Social Abilities	____(25)		____(100)
	Interactional Abilities	____(53)		____(100)
	Interpretive Abilities	____(34)		____(100)
	TOTAL	____(151)		____(100)

SELF CARE ABILITIES

1. Voluntary Movements

	Yes (1)	No (0)
(a) *Lips:* maintains relaxation of the lips when light pressure is applied in the form of a tongue blade or flexed finger moved along the lips Score	____	____
(b) *Fingers:* maintains finger extension when the examiner stimulates the palm of the open hand with a finger Score	____	____
(c) *Arms:* passively extends the arm to some extent after each of four times that the examiner bends and extends the person's arms Score	____	____
Subtotal (1. a-c)	____	(3)

2. Spatial Orientation

(a) Right/Left Orientation
Ask person to demonstrate awareness of left and right orientation in simple (single), complex (in combination), or other (another person) levels:

---

*Copyrighted by Dawson, Wells, & Kline (1993).

		Yes (1)	No (0)	
Single:	(i) touch your right hand	——	——	
	(ii) touch your left foot	——	——	
Complex:	(i) touch your right ear with your left hand	——	——	
	(ii) point to your left eye with your right hand	——	——	
Other				
Person:	(i) touch my left hand	——	——	
	(ii) touch my right hand	——	——	
	Score		——	(6)

(b) *Point of Origin*
Is able to return to room/home
without assistance (i.e., finding own room) —— ——

                                          Score —— (1)

                                     Subtotal —— **(7)**
                                     (2. a-b)

3. Purposeful Movements

(a) *Initiation and Follow-Through*
    (i) Show three objects (e.g., pen, spoon,
    soap) to individual and ask him/her to
    show you how to use them - if done correctly —— (3)
    score three for each correct answer. If done —— (3)
    incorrectly, proceed to. —— (3)

    (ii) Demonstrate the use of the objects and ask the —— (2)
    person to copy your actions. Score two for each cor- —— (2)
    rect answer. If done *incorrectly*, proceed to: —— (2)

    (iii) Place the objects (one at a time) in person's —— (1)
    hand and ask patient to pretend to use them. —— (1)
    Score one for each correct answer. —— (1)
                               Score —— (9)

(b) *Simple Activity*
Individual performs 2 simple tasks using "one" object.

	Yes (1)	No (0)	
(i) Instruct individual to comb hair:			
initiates activity	——	——	
follows through activity by self	——	——	
completes activity by self	——	——	
stops activity by self	——	——	
sequences activity properly (i.e., in right order)	——	——	
(ii) Instruct individual to drink from a cup:			
initiates activity	——	——	
follows through activity by self	——	——	
completes activity by self	——	——	
stops activity by self	——	——	
sequences activity properly (i.e., in right order)	——	——	
Score		——	(10)

(c) *Complex Activity*
Individual performs 2 complex tasks that require using more than one object.

	Yes (1)	No (0)
(i) Instruct individual to wash hands using a washcloth and soap:		
initiates activity	___	___
follows through activity by self	___	___
completes activity by self	___	___
stops activity by self	___	___
sequences activity properly (i.e., in right order)	___	___
(ii) Instruct individual to put on socks and shoes:		
initiates activity	___	___
follows through activity by self	___	___
completes activity by self	___	___
stops activity by self	___	___
sequences activity properly (i.e., in right order)	___	___

Score	___	(10)
Subtotal 3.a-c	___	**(29)**

SELF-CARE ABILITIES SCORE

(a) **Total score achieved = __**
(add subtotals)
(b) **Total score possible = <u>39</u>**
(c) **% Score = <u> (a) </u> x 100**
   (b)

SOCIAL ABILITIES

1. To Give and Receive Attention

(a) Greet individual with "hello" or "good morning."
Response is *one* of the following:

(i) verbal reply	___	(4)
(ii) smile only	___	(3)
(iii) eye contact only	___	(2)
(iv) mutters	___	(1)
(v) no change in behavior to suggest response	___	(0)
Score	___	(4)

(b) Initiate a handshake (i.e., offer your hand to the person).
Response is *one* of the following:

(i) grasps offered hand (self-initiated)	___	(3)
(ii) other initiated (you take his/her hand)	___	(2)
(iii) initiates letting go	___	(1)
(iv) no response	___	(0)
Score	___	(3)

(c) Individual's response to "how are you?" is *one* of the following:

    (i) verbal reply   ____ (3)

    (ii) verbal but unclear   ____ (2)

    (iii) non-verbal (eye gaze, nod, smile)   ____ (1)

    (iv) no change in behavior to suggest response   ____ (0)

                        Score   ____ (3)

(d) Address individual by name and give your name.
Response is *one* of the following:

    (i) verbal reply   ____ (4)

    (ii) facial responses (nods, smiles, looks)   ____ (3)

    (iii) body language response (leans toward)   ____ (2)

    (iv) mumbles   ____ (1)

    (v) no response   ____ (0)

                     Score   ____ (4)

                     Subtotal   ____ **(14)**

                     (1. a-d)

2. To Engage/Participate in Conversation

Initiate a topic of conversation with the individual. Response
is *one* from topic and verbal, and *one* from nonverbal.

(a) *Topic*

    Stays on topic   ____ (2)

    Relates improbable events   ____ (1)

    No response to topic   ____ (0)

                 Score   ____ (2)

(b) *Verbal*

    Distinct verbal response   ____ (2)

    Indistinct verbal response   ____ (1)

    No verbal response   ____ (0)

                 Score   ____ (2)

(c) *Nonverbal*

    Takes turns, looks, listens or nods   ____ (1)

    No response   ____ (0)

                 Score   ____ (1)

                 Subtotal   ____ **(5)**

                 (2. a-c)

3. Humor Appreciation

(a) Inform individual that you have a cartoon you would
like to show him/her. Show cartoon. Response is *one* of
the following:

    Laughs out loud or makes relevant comments   ____ (3)

    Laughs quietly   ____ (2)

    Smiles   ____ (1)

    No response   ____ (0)

                     Score   ____ (3)

(b) Inform individual that you have a joke you would like to tell him/her. Tell a *short* joke which is non-prejudicial and non-controversial. Keep a straight face at the punch line. Example: "A kangaroo walked into a bar and asked the bartender for a beer. The bartender gave the kangaroo a beer and said, 'That'll be 5 dollars.' Later the bartender returned and said, 'We don't get many kangaroos in here.' The kangaroo said, 'I'm not surprised, at these prices.'" Response is *one* of the following:

Laughs at punch line or makes relevant comments	____	(3)
Changes facial expression at punch line	____	(2)
Unexpected response at punch line (e.g., crying, anger, etc.)	____	(1)
No response	____	(0)
Score	____	(3)
Subtotal	____	**(6)**
(3. a-b)		

SOCIAL ABILITIES SCORE

(a) **Total score achieved = ____**
   (add subtotals)
(b) **Total score possible = 25**
(c) **% Score = (a) x 100**
              (b)

INTERACTIONAL ABILITIES

1. Comprehension Abilities

(a) *Understanding of Commands*

	Yes (1)	No (0)
(i) One-Part—Self		
Ask individual to follow four, 1-part (1 verb, 1 noun) commands relating to self:		
Touch your nose	____	____
Raise your arms	____	____
Point to your feet	____	____
Close your eyes	____	____
(ii) One-Part—Object		
Ask individual to follow four, 1-part (1 verb, 1 noun) commands relating to objects:		
Point to the ceiling	____	____
Open the book	____	____
Touch the chair	____	____
Pick up the cup	____	____

(iii) Two-Part—Self
Ask individual to follow three, 2-part (2 verbs, 2 nouns) commands relating to self:

	Yes (1)	No (0)
Stamp your feet and then close your eyes	___	___
Touch your cheek and then pat your head	___	___
Blow through your lips and then point to your teeth	___	___

(iv) Two-Part—Object
Ask individual to follow three, 2-part (2 verbs, 2 nouns) commands relating to objects:

Give me the pen, then point to the window	___	___
Touch the chair and point to the bed	___	___
Look at the floor and touch my ring	___	___

(v) Three-Part—Simple
Ask individual to follow *two* simple (1 verb, 3 nouns) 3-part commands:

Point to your knees, then point to your head, then point to your stomach	___	___
Pick up the pen, pick up the cloth, and then pick up the spoon	___	___

(vi) Three-Part-Complex
Direct individual to follow *two* complex (3 verbs, 3 nouns) 3-part commands:

Point to my face, raise your arms, and clap your hands	___	___
Put your hands on the chair arms, slide your bottom forward, and stand on your feet	___	___
Score	___	(18)

(b) *Reading Comprehension*
For the following, show the individual written commands of increasing complexity (1-part to 3-part commands). Each command should be on a separate page or card and be written large enough for the person to see. Present one at a time. Ask the individual to follow through on the written command. Then ask the person to read the command aloud.

(i) One-Part
Ask individual to follow through on three 1-part commands. Ask the person to read the command aloud:

	Follow through (1)	No (0)	Read (1)	No (0)
Point to the ceiling	___	___	___	___
Touch my arm	___	___	___	___
Hand me the pen	___	___	___	___

(ii) Two-Part
Repeat and score for three 2-part written commands:

Raise your arm(s) and close your eyes	___	___	___	___
Point to the ceiling and touch my arm	___	___	___	___
Grasp the arms of the chair and turn your head	___	___	___	___

(iii) Three-Part

Repeat and score for two 3-part written commands:

Point to the floor, touch the arm of the
chair and then take my hand   ____ ____ ____ ____

Put your hands on your knees, look at
me and count to three   ____ ____ ____ ____

        Score:

        Follow through ____ (8) + Read ____ (8) = ____ (16)

        Subtotal   ____ **(34)**

        (1. a-b)

2. Expression Abilities

(a) *Verbal Object Identification*

Use four objects, which are familiar and seen daily, e.g., pen, comb, fork, spoon. Each is held up and the person is asked to name the object.

	Yes (1)	No (0)
	____	____
	____	____
	____	____
Score		____ (4)

(b) *Word Retrieval*

Completes the last word of four familiar sentences:

	Yes	No
The grass is ____ (green)	____	____
Ice is ____ (cold)	____	____
Violets are ____ (blue)	____	____
They fought like cats and ____ (dogs)	____	____
Score		____ (4)

(c) *Description*

Ask the individual to describe the room in which the assessment is taking place:

Description includes 4 or more objects (including
floor, ceiling, walls) used in sentence form   ____ (5)

Description includes 4 or more objects but sentences
are incomplete   ____ (4)

Description includes less than 4 objects but they are
correct   ____ (3)

Description includes less than 4 objects but they are
incorrect   ____ (2)

Verbal response attempted but no object words used   ____ (1)

No response or verbal reaction   ____ (0)

        Score   ____ (5)

(d) *Written Expression*

(i) Show individual an object and ask individual to
write its name: e.g., cup, pen, book:

	Yes (1)	No (0)
	____	____
	____	____
	____	____

(ii) Show the individual three familiar objects and   Yes   No
ask him/her to write what these objects are used   (1)   (0)
for: e.g., to drink, to write, to read   ____   ____
                                                        ____   ____
                                                        ____   ____

                                      Score   ____   (6)
                                      Subtotal   ____   **(19)**
                                      (2. a-d)

INTERACTIONAL ABILITIES SCORE

(a) **Total score achieved = ____**
    (add subtotals)
(b) **Total score possible = 53**
(c) **% Score = (a) x 100**
          (b)

INTERPRETIVE ABILITIES

1. Recognition

(a) *Self-Recognition*   Yes   No
                                                        (1)   (0)
   (i) identifies self in mirror   ____   ____
   (ii) ask person to read her/his own name and then
   ask whose name it is   ____   ____
                                      Score   ____   (2)

(b) *Facial Affect Recognition*
   Inform individual that you would like him/her to
   tell you how the person in the picture is feeling by
   the expression on his/her face. Record description.
   If no verbal description, ask individual to choose if
   facial expression is sad, angry or happy.
   (i) sad   ____   ____
   (ii) angry   ____   ____
   (iii) happy   ____   ____
                                      Score   ____   (3)

(c) *Object Recognition by Touch*
   (i) Ask individual to close eyes and identify 4 small   ____   ____
   objects placed in hand, one at a time by touch   ____   ____
   (e.g., comb, ring, key, spoon, or fork).   ____   ____
                                                           ____   ____

   (ii) Ask individual to close eyes. Put large cup in
   one hand and a small cup in the other. Ask
   individual to identify the hand holding the larger cup. ____   ____
                                      Score   ____   (5)

(d) *Recognition of Time*
   (i) *Clock*
   Show individual a drawing of a clock showing a
   specific on-the-hour time and ask the person to say
   what time is indicated on the clock.   ____   ____

Show individual a drawing of a clock showing hour
and minute time and ask the person to say what
time is indicated on the clock.   ____ ____

Score   ____ (2)

(ii) *Date*
Show individual a monthly calendar and ask to
point out two dates.   ____ ____

                                                         ____ ____

Point to two dates on a monthly calendar and ask
individual to read these dates.   ____ ____

                                                         ____ ____

Score   ____ (4)
Subtotal   ____ **(16)**
(1. a-d)

2. *Recall*

(a) Recall of familiar objects and places (F.A.C.T. test).
Ask individual to recall as many fruits as possible. Repeat for animals,
colors, and towns

	3 (8-10 Items)	2 (5-7)	1 (1-4)	0 (0)
Fruits	____	____	____	____
Animals	____	____	____	____
Colors	____	____	____	____
Towns	____	____	____	____

Score   (12)
Subtotal   ____ **(12)**

3. Feeling States

(a) *Subjective*
Inform the individual that you would like to talk with him/her
about how he/she has been feeling in the last week. When
asking the following questions, it may be necessary to preface
with probes (e.g., "Do you have feelings now of ____?" or
"Have you ever had feelings of ____?"
(i) sadness (no)   ____
(ii) anxiety (no)   ____
(iii) happiness (yes)   ____
(iv) worry (no)   ____
(v) contentment (yes)   ____
(vi) boredom (no)   ____

Score 1 if answers given are as shown. Score 0 if answers
given are not shown

Score   ____ (6)
Subtotal   ____ **(6)**

(b) Depression
Suspect depression if the individual expresses no to (iii) and
(v) and yes to (i) (ii) (iv) and (vi). Refer to doctor.

INTERPRETIVE ABILITIES SCORE

     (a) Total score achieved = ____
         (add subtotals)
     (b) Total score possible = <u>34</u>
     (c) % Score = <u>(a)</u> x 100
               (b)

FINAL SCORE   ____

Total Possible Score   (151)
% of total possible score ____

5

The Family Well-Being Assessment Tool

Shirley M. Caldwell

This chapter discusses the Family Well-Being Assessment Tool, a measure of family well-being.

PURPOSE

The Family Well-Being Assessment (FWA) is an instrument designed to measure various aspects of family life on a continuum from well-being to stress. An earlier version of this instrument was called Family Stress Assessment and was used in an investigative study in 1983 (Caldwell, 1983). The present version has been refined through work done for the University of Maryland's Measurement of Clinical and Educational Nursing Outcomes Project. The instrument uses a 6–point Likert scale, with low scores demonstrating less stress or a greater perception of well-being.

The conceptual model for the FWA was begun by Thomas (1981), whose beginning theory of family stress I have adapted and expanded with his permission, since it was generally consistent with my concept of family stress/well-being. Thomas proposed that family stress research should be conceptualized by assessing family structural components, the family function or roles, and individual and family vulnerability. In the past, family stress research focused on isolated aspects of the total picture. Although selected traits of the relationship of parents and children have been investigated extensively, such relationships are almost always dealt with out of context, as if the family as a whole did not exist. It is my belief that a family is an interactional system of two or more members in the process of, or at the level of, defining the nature of their kinship or intimate relationship, which is in agreement with Watzlawick, Beavin, & Jackson (1967). The FWA attempts to assess family as an interactional system based on Thomas's work and on my conception of family stress/well-being.

THEORETICAL BASIS

The FWA instrument views the family as a social system (Katz & Kahn, 1966; Miller, 1971). The family is believed to be the primary influence on the behavior and experience of each individual member. What affects one member of the family has an impact on the other family members (Sabbeth, 1984). Thus, members must adapt to stressors from other parts of the system as well as to stress that is self-generated. Conversely, the sense of well-being of one member has an effect on other members.

Thomas's (1981) conceptual model defines the family system as (1) the relationship of structure, the units of which the family is composed; (2) the interrelationship of function or roles in the way the family tasks are done; and (3) the vulnerability to other influences such as those of genetic, physiological, sociological, or psychological origin. This basic definition was used and expanded on to produce the following components that describe the FWA instrument. These are: (1) family structural components—family stress, family satisfaction, family support, family cohesion, and family adaptation; (2) family functional role processes—role conflict, role overload, role ambiguity, role nonparticipation, and role preparedness; and (3) family vulnerability—psychosomatic symptoms and life satisfaction.

If the concept of multiple, interactional factors is valid, then it is essential to develop a model identifying the component parts and their dynamic relationship to family stress/well-being. Using this model, the FWA instrument can measure these component parts and lead us to a greater understanding of the influence of these components on the individual member and the family as a whole. From this knowledge, we can then make more appropriate family interventions to decrease stress and increase family health.

The central claim of this model is that the family is responsible for creating and maintaining a physical, emotional, social, and spiritual environment that will preserve and enhance the well-being of its members. Family pathology is predicted on the assumption that family structure, functional role processes, and vulnerability are significant factors in the predisposition, inception, and maintenance of many diseases and overall family stress.

In essence, family structure, role process, and vulnerability and the disease processes are elements of an open system (Miller, 1971; von Bertalanffy, 1968). Biochemical, physiological, psychological, social, and spiritual systems interact to transmit stress throughout the system. Family well-being is threatened. However, an existing dysfunctional system of family structure, role process, and vulnerability has a strong independent influence on the development and maintenance of illness within family members. Pratt's (1976) findings suggest that it is not simply a number of separate factors that affect health, but it is the family's overall pattern of arrangements for relating to and working with each other that is important.

Family structure, functional role process, and vulnerability are by no means novel concepts in the study of family systems and health. Their novelty and uniqueness are attributable to their placement in a dynamic, multidimensional model (see Figure 5.1) that posits an interaction between the components as necessary (versus exclusive) dimensions in the analysis of family well-being. It should be emphasized that the combination of stressors, family structure, functional role processes, and vulnerability are not the sole cause of any specific disease state. Nuckolls (1975) believed that instead of searching for a specific relationship, it is perhaps more useful to view factors as detractors or enhancers of overall health or as interacting contributors to both the susceptibility to and prognosis of disease in general. The factors may account for a sizable portion of the etiology and pathology, but they do not by themselves account for a particular health outcome. Perhaps they are best conceptualized as predictors of increased risk.

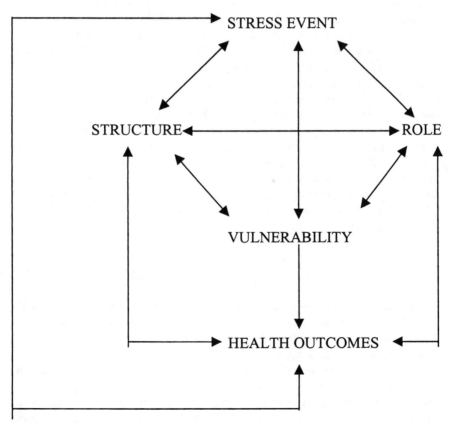

FIGURE 5.1 Model for family well-being.

The FWA has thus been developed on the basis of a conceptual framework of interrelated and interdependent concepts applicable to family well-being, and appears capable of assessing family well-being using these concepts (Caldwell, 1983; Caldwell & Pichert, 1985; Pettegrew et al., 1980). What remains to be demonstrated is the configuration and strength of the relationship between family structural components and functional role process, vulnerability, and state of family health.

The conceptual framework that has been developed provides a mapping sentence. A mapping sentence serves two functions in relation to theory building. It allows the researcher to articulate visually the elements of the construct under investigation. It also provides a means of identifying specific facets of the construct, the components of which can be expanded or modified to extend and enrich the theory and improve the measuring instrument (Elizur, 1970; McCubbin et al., 1980). Embedded within this framework is a mandate for research scholars to turn their attention to the entire family as an important unit of study. The following mapping sentence of family well-being is offered to demonstrate the hypothesized relationship of stress, family structure, functional role processes, and vulnerability to family well-being.

The FWA is the norm-referenced cognitive assessment by members of a nuclear family of their perceptions of the extent to which the following are present in family life: (1) family structural components—family stress, family satisfaction, family support, family cohesion, and family adaptation; (2) family functional role processes—role conflict, role overload, role ambiguity, role nonparticipation, and role preparedness; and (3) family vulnerability—psychosomatic symptoms and life satisfaction.

The components of the mapping sentence are indicators of family stress or well-being, ranging from very strong to very weak manifestations on each item. If these measures of family stress can identify families at high risk, then intervention and treatment strategies can be developed to decrease or control those factors causing family stress (based on Thomas' 1981 conceptual model).

ADMINISTRATION AND SCORING

Individual family members rate each item of family well-being on a 6-point Likert scale ranging from STRONG agreement through Moderate agreement, slight agreement, slight disagreement, and Moderate disagreement to STRONG disagreement.

There are two versions of the test: a shorter 45–item test for children 9 to 18 years of age (10 subscales) and a longer 57–item test for parents (11 subscales). See appendices to this chapter for the tests. The time required to complete the test is 15 to 20 minutes. All items are measured on a 6–point Likert-type scale, scored from 1 to 6, with 1 being most desirable. The number of items in each subscale varies from three to eight. Some items require reverse coding. A total Well-Being score is obtained by summing the average score of each subscale. The total possible range is 11 to 66. A low score indicates well-being or low stress. Item numbers on the children's version of the instrument are not consecutive but match similar items on the parent's version so that differences can be more easily identified for individual families. An SPSS computer program is available for computer scoring.

RELIABILITY AND VALIDITY

Reliability

Reliability, (Waltz, Strickland, & Lenz, 1984), was assessed in four ways:

1. Item analysis, was performed. Items were deleted if they detracted from the subscale alpha by more than 4. None of the deleted items is included in the current instrument.
2. A correlational matrix was run. Items with extremely high (>.88) or low (primarily negative) correlations were deleted.
3. Internal consistency, using Cronbach's alpha, has been done twice, once in 1985 using original data (Caldwell, 1983). Inappropriate terms (i.e., items that had two ideas) were deleted so that alpha values ranged from .37 to .86 for the subscales. Cronbach's alphas were recomputed in 1986, using the revised instrument and the data from the increased sample size of 204 children and 185 parents. The number of items per subscale varies from 3 to 8, so the subscales were considered worthwhile for this stage of instrument development. Overall instrument reliability was .89 for the children's version and .90 for the parents'.
4. Test-retest, was conducted using 11 families (*N* = 82), with a retest time of 1 to 3 weeks, It was found to be .88.

Validity

The validity of the instrument, (Waltz et al., 1984), was assessed three ways:

1. Face validity is not a stringent method of assessing validity. However, because the instrument was developed from a conceptual framework, each of the items for the subscales was developed from the definition.
2. Content validity was assessed by two specialists, Ora Strickland, who at the time was Doctoral Program Evaluator, University of Maryland, and

Linda Cronenwett, who at the time was Director of Nursing Research, Dartmouth Hitchcock Medical Center, Hanover, NH, each with a special interest in family research. Their interrater agreement or Content Validity Index for each of the subscales ranged from .9 to 1. Items were rated from 1 *not relevant* to 4 *very relevant*. Items rated 3 or 4 were retained. Those rated 1 or 2 were deleted.

3. Construct validity is of greatest importance when testing the affective domain. Previous research using contrasting groups found the instrument was able to separate high-stress persons from low-stress persons (Pettegrew et al., 1980) and high-stress families from low stress families (Caldwell & Pichert, 1985).

Construct validity was further supported when data from families without a chronically ill child, (Keys, 1986; Yeagley, 1985), hypothesized to have lower stress, were compared to data from families with a chronically ill child (Caldwell & Pichert, 1985; Chandler, 1985). Parents showed a greater difference than children.

Data from parents of chronically ill children were compared to data from parents of children not chronically ill ($N = 91$). The t-tests for individual subscale differences and the total overall instrument scores demonstrated less stress or a greater perception of well-being for parents of the children not chronically ill. The findings were statistically significant at $p < .01$ for six of the subscales, at $p < .05$ for two more, and not statistically significant for Family Adaptation, Role Overload, and Role Preparedness. Role Conflict difference is reported at $p < .06$. The level of significance for differences between the two groups using the total instrument was $p < .01$.

Children's perceptions were found to be less different. For each subscale, and the total score, children from families without a chronically ill child ($N = 98$) perceived less stress than did children from families that included a chronically ill child ($N = 110$). The C-test for difference was statistically significant ($p < .05$) for three subscales—Family Adaptation, Family Stress, and Family Satisfaction—and $p < .01$ for Psychosomatic Symptoms and Role Nonparticipation. The level of significance for difference between the two groups using the total instrument was $p < .05$).

CONCLUSIONS AND RECOMMENDATIONS

The FWA instrument was used in a 2-year follow-up study of families previously studied by Caldwell (1986) and was found to be a sensitive instrument for measuring individual and family stress. By using the subscales, researchers are able to better understand how the major sources of perceived stress vary for individual family members. Two major grants have been written that will include further use of the instrument in assessing individual and family well-being or stress.

Three graduate students also used the FWA instrument. Yeagley (1985) looked at stress differences between families who used the birthing room experience versus families who used the traditional labor and delivery experience. No significant differences were found between the two groups of families. Chandler (1985) measured stress in families with a child with cancer and compared results to the children with diabetes studies by Caldwell (1986). No significant differences in total stress were found between the two groups; however, family stress (FSt) was perceived as higher by children with cancer than by children with diabetes. In addition, both children with cancer and their siblings experienced more psychosomatic symptoms (PS) such as headaches and stomach upsets than did children in the diabetes group. Keys (1986) measured stress in families that have no chronically ill children. These measures are being compared to the measures obtained for children from families with diabetic children. These analyses have not been completed. The FWA instrument has also been found to be sensitive to individual differences in the same family (Caldwell, 1983).

The author and a cotherapist need results from the instrument to provide direction for family counseling in families that have a child newly diagnosed with insulin-dependent diabetes. The use of this instrument can provide health care providers and family counselors with increased information about the family that will aid them in identifying areas at risk so that appropriate interventions can be implemented. The anticipated result would be a healthier family system requiring fewer health care provider visits or family counseling sessions.

REFERENCES

Caldwell, S. M. (1983). *Family communication patterns, siblings, and insulin dependent diabetic children.* Unpublished doctoral dissertation, Vanderbilt University, Nashville, TN.

Caldwell, S. M. (1986). Systems theory applied to families with insulin-dependent diabetic children. In S. Stinson, J. C. Kerr, P. Giovannetti, P. Field, & J. MacPhail (Eds.), *Proceedings: International Nursing Research Conference* (p. 85). Edmonton, Alberta: University of Alberta Press.

Caldwell, S. M. (1988). Measuring family well-being: Conceptual model, reliability, validity, and use. In C. F. Waltz & O. L. Strickland (Eds.), *Measurement of nursing outcomes: Vol. 1: Measuring client outcomes* (pp. 287–308). New York: Springer Publishing Co.

Caldwell, S. M., & Pichert, J. W. (1985). Systems theory applied to families with a diabetic child. *Family Systems Medicine, 3*(1), 34–44.

Chandler, D. L. (1985). *Stress and self-concepts of chronically ill children and their healthy siblings.* Unpublished master's thesis, Vanderbilt University, Nashville, TN.

Elizur, D. (1970). *Adapting to innovation.* Jerusalem: Jerusalem Academic Press.

Katz, D., & Kahn, R. L. (1966). *The social psychology of organizations.* New York: Wiley.

Keys, J. E. (1986). *A comparison of perceived stress and self-concept measures for children from families with and without chronically ill children.* Unpublished raw data.

McCubbin, H., Joy, C., Cauble, E., Corneau, J., Patterson, J., & Needle, R. (1980). Family stress and coping: A decade review. *Journal of Marriage and the Family, 42*(4), 125–141.

Miller, J. C. (1971). Systems theory and family psychotherapy. *Nursing Clinics of North America, 6*(3), 395–406.

Nuckolls, K. B. (1975). Life crisis and psychosocial assets: Some clinical applications. In B. H. Kaplan & J. Cassel (Eds.), *Family and health: An epidemiological approach.* (pp. 39–62). Chapel Hill, NC: University of North Carolina, Institute for Social Science Research.

Pettegrew, L., Thomas, R. C., Costello, D. E., Wolf, G. E., Lennox, L., & Thomas, S. L. (1980). Job related stress in a medical center organization: Management of communication issues. In D. Nimmo (Ed.), *Communication yearbook,* 4 (pp. 625–653). New Brunswick, NJ: Transaction.

Pratt, L. (1976). An exploration of the dynamics of the overlapping worlds of work and family. *Family Process, 15,* 143–165.

Sabbeth, B. (1984). Understanding the impact of chronic childhood illness on families. *Pediatric Clinics of North America, 31*(1), 47–57.

Thomas, R. C. (1981, May). *Conceptual foundation for a theoretical model of family well-being.* Paper presented at the convention of the Health Communications Division of the International Communication Association, Minneapolis.

von Bertalanffy, L. (1968). *General systems theory.* New York: George Braziller.

Waltz, C., Strickland, O., & Lenz, E. (1984). *Measurement in nursing research.* Philadelphia: F. A. Davis.

Watzlawick, P., Beavin, J., & Jackson, D. (1967). *Pragmatics of human communication.* New York: Norton.

Yeagley, S. C. (1985). *Siblings at birth: Long term stress effects.* Unpublished master's thesis, Vanderbilt University, Nashville, TN.

APPENDIX A: FAMILY WELL-BEING ASSESSMENT—PARENT

There is much about how families work together and support each other that researchers don't understand. The following questions concern what it is like to be a member of your family. Please answer each question as honestly as possible but don't spend too much time on any one question. All questions pertain to *your role as a parent*. All of your answers *will remain anonymous*.

There are two sections in this questionnaire. Each section will have slightly different answer categories. Before beginning each section, please read the answer categories for that section very carefully, and then proceed by *circling* the answer that best represents your particular *feelings*.

In this section the following scale is used for all questions. Circle the answer that best suits your agreement or disagreement with the statement.

YES = STRONG Agreement
Yes = Moderate agreement
yes = slight agreement
no = slight disagreement
No = Moderate disagreement
NO = STRONG Disagreement

1. At times I cannot get my work done without
   doing things that my spouse disagrees with. *YES* Yes yes no No *NO*
2. I know what my family expects of me as a
   parent from one day to the next. *YES* Yes yes no No *NO*
3. Most of the time other family members
   expect me to be a better parent. *YES* Yes yes no No *NO*
4. My family regularly takes time to discuss
   family issues. *YES* Yes yes no No *NO*
5. There is a lot of strain on the members of
   our family. *YES* Yes yes no No *NO*
6. In general, my family is the kind of family
   I want to be a member of. *YES* Yes yes no No *NO*
7. My life is currently very rewarding. *YES* Yes yes no No *NO*
8. I have a hard time satisfying the conflicting
   demands of the members of my family. *YES* Yes yes no No *NO*
9. I am sure what my family expects of me. *YES* Yes yes no No *NO*
11. My family expects me to do more at home
    than I am able to do. *YES* Yes yes no No *NO*
12. I have influence over what happens in my
    family. *YES* Yes yes no No *NO*
14. My spouse understands that I need to have
    time alone with my friends. *YES* Yes yes no No *NO*

15. I currently find my life very hopeful.   *YES* Yes yes no No *NO*
16. I would definitely say that my home is a
    stressful place for family members to live.   *YES* Yes yes no No *NO*
17. I am extremely satisfied with my role as a
    parent.   *YES* Yes yes no No *NO*
18. I currently find my life quite lonely.   *YES* Yes yes no No *NO*
19. There is a difference between the way my
    spouse thinks things should be done and
    the way I think they should be done.   *YES* Yes yes no No *NO*
21. I receive enough information to effectively
    carry out my duties as a parent.   *YES* Yes yes no No *NO*
22. Even when we are not together as a family,
    I have a sense of family support.   *YES* Yes yes no No *NO*
26. My life is currently quite empty.   *YES* Yes yes no No *NO*
27. My job as a parent is extremely fulfilling in
    comparison to other interests in my life.   *YES* Yes yes no No *NO*
30. Other family members feel I am a very
    capable parent.   *YES* Yes yes no No *NO*
31. I ask other family members questions,
    and I often do what they suggest.   *YES* Yes yes no No *NO*
32. In my family I don't really know what my
    family thinks of me.   *YES* Yes yes no No *NO*
33. I would describe my home as a tightly
    wound spring ready to explode.   *YES* Yes yes no No *NO*
34. Family rules change as children get older.   *YES* Yes yes no No *NO*
35. Most of my friends are friends of the family.   *YES* Yes yes no No *NO*
36. My family rarely does anything together
    for fun.   *YES* Yes yes no No *NO*
38. I listen carefully to other family members
    and react in such a way that they know I
    am listening to them.   *YES* Yes yes no No *NO*
39. I have too many responsibilities at home.   *YES* Yes yes no No *NO*
40. My training to be a parent was inadequate in
    preparing me for the daily demands of
    parenting.   *YES* Yes yes no No *NO*
41. I currently find my life very enjoyable.   *YES* Yes yes no No *NO*
42. Family decisions are made regardless of
    my opinion.   *YES* Yes yes no No *NO*
44. I adapt quickly to new situations in my family.   *YES* Yes yes no No *NO*
45. My role as a parent interferes with other
    roles in my life.   *YES* Yes yes no No *NO*
46. Child discipline is handled mostly by one
    parent/adult in this family.   *YES* Yes yes no No *NO*
47. At home, I have extra work beyond what
    should be expected of me.   *YES* Yes yes no No *NO*

49. I am prepared to handle most situations
    that I encounter within my family   *YES* Yes yes no No *NO*
50. I receive conflicting requests from
    different members of my family.   *YES* Yes yes no No *NO*
52. When asked, I am able to tell someone
    what is included in my role as a parent.   *YES* Yes yes no No *NO*

The following section contains questions which describe your and your family's reactions related to situations at home. Please indicate the extent to which each question applies to your family situation by *circling* the most appropriate point on the scale.

YES	=	Almost *always*
Yes	=	Very often
yes	=	Frequently
no	=	0ccasionally
No	=	Not very often
NO	=	Almost *never*

54. I experience stomach upsets.   *YES* Yes yes no No *NO*
55. My spouse supports me and my decisions in
    front of other family members and friends. *YES* Yes yes no No *NO*
56. I have trouble getting to sleep or staying
    asleep.   *YES* Yes yes no No *NO*
57. My family pays attention to what I am
    saying.   *YES* Yes yes no No *NO*
59. I am troubled by headaches.   *YES* Yes yes no No *NO*
60. I worry a great deal about my family.   *YES* Yes yes no No *NO*
62. My family members stand up for each
    other to outsiders.   *YES* Yes yes no No *NO*
63. I am bothered by nervousness, feeling
    fidgety or tense.   *YES* Yes yes no No *NO*
65. I have had a recent loss or gain of weight *YES* Yes yes no No *NO*
66. When I really need to talk with someone,
    the children in my family are willing to
    listen.   *YES* Yes yes no No *NO*
67. My spouse pays attention to what I are
    saying.   *YES* Yes yes no No *NO*
68. When I really need to talk to my spouse
    s/he is willing to listen.   *YES* Yes yes no No *NO*
69. If I choose to do things differently than
    family custom, this would create a lot of
    family tension.   *YES* Yes yes no No *NO*
71. My family asks my opinion on important
    matters.   *YES* Yes yes no No *NO*

72. I feel I am unprepared to do my job as a
    parent.   *YES* Yes yes no No *NO*
73. I am told about important things that are
    happening with my family.   *YES* Yes yes no No *NO*
74. I am unsure of what all my responsibilities
    are as a parent.   *YES* Yes yes no No *NO*

APPENDIX B: FAMILY WELL-BEING ASSESSMENT—CHILD

There is much about how families work together and support each other
that researchers don't understand. The following questions concern what
it is like to be a member of your family. Please answer each question as
honestly as possible but don't spend too much time on any one question.
All questions pertain to you as a child. *All of your answers will remain
anonymous.*

There are two sections in this questionnaire. Each section will have
slightly different answer categories. Before beginning each section, please
read the answer categories for that section very carefully, and then proceed
by *circling* the answer that best represents your particular feelings.

In this section the following scale is used for all questions. Circle the
answer that best suits your agreement or disagreement with the statement.

> *YES* – STRONG Agreement
> Yes = Moderate agreement
> yes = slight agreement
> no = slight disagreement
> No = Moderate disagreement
> *NO* = STRONG Disagreement

1. I am asked to do things around my home.   *YES* Yes yes no No *NO*
2. I know what my family expects of me as a
   child from one day to the next.   *YES* Yes yes no No *NO*
3. Most of the time other family members
   expect me to be a better child.   *YES* Yes yes no No *NO*
4. My family regularly takes time to discuss
   family matters.   *YES* Yes yes no No *NO*
5. There is a lot of tenseness, pressure on
   the members of our family.   *YES* Yes yes no No *NO*
6. My family is the kind of family I want to
   be a member of.   *YES* Yes yes no No *NO*
7. My life right now is very happy.   *YES* Yes yes no No *NO*
8. I have a hard time pleasing my parents
   because they each expect different things
   from me.   *YES* Yes yes no No *NO*

9. I am sure of what my family expects of me. *YES* Yes yes no No *NO*
11. My family expects me to do more at home
    than I am able to do. *YES* Yes yes no No *NO*
12. What I think can change what happens in
    my family. *YES* Yes yes no No *NO*
13. I am allowed to make more personal
    decisions now than a year ago. *YES* Yes yes no No *NO*
14. My family recognizes the value of private
    time for each member. *YES* Yes yes no No *NO*
15. I look forward to living my life. *YES* Yes yes no No *NO*
16. I would definitely say that my home is a
    stressful place for family members to live. *YES* Yes yes no No *NO*
17. All in all, I would say I am extremely satis-
    fied with being a member in this family. *YES* Yes yes no No *NO*
18. I currently find my life quite lonely. *YES* Yes yes no No *NO*
19. There is a difference between the way my
    parents think things should be done. *YES* Yes yes no No *NO*
21. I get enough direction to know what is
    expected of me as a child in our family. *YES* Yes yes no No *NO*
22. Even when I am away from my family, I
    know they are interested in what I am
    doing. *YES* Yes yes no No *NO*
26. My life is really quite empty. *YES* Yes yes no No *NO*
27. Being a member in this family is very
    important to me compared with friend-
    ships outside of my home. *YES* Yes yes no No *NO*
31. I ask other family members questions and
    I often do what they suggest. *YES* Yes yes no No *NO*
32. I don't really know what my family thinks
    of me. *YES* Yes yes no No *NO*
33. I would describe my home as a stressful
    place to live. *YES* Yes yes no No *NO*
35. Most of my friends are friends of the
    entire family. *YES* Yes yes no No *NO*
36. My family rarely does anything together
    for fun. *YES* Yes yes no No *NO*
38. I listen very carefully to my parents so
    they know I am listening to them. *YES* Yes yes no No *NO*
39. I have too many responsibilities at home. *YES* Yes yes no No *NO*
41. My life right now is very enjoyable. *YES* Yes yes no No *NO*
42. In my home, I feel that it is useless for
    me to make suggestions regarding family
    issues. *YES* Yes yes no No *NO*

The following section contains questions that describe your and your family's reactions related to situations at home. Please indicate the extent to which each question applies to your family situation by circling the most appropriate point on the scale.

YES	=	Almost *always*
Yes	=	Very often
yes	=	Frequently
no	=	0ccasionally
No	=	Not very often
NO	=	Almost *never*

53. When I really need to talk to my mother, she is willing to listen.   *YES* Yes yes no No *NO*
54. I have stomach upsets.   *YES* Yes yes no No *NO*
55. My parents support me and my decisions in front of other family members and friends.   *YES* Yes yes no No *NO*
56. I have trouble getting to sleep or staying asleep.   *YES* Yes yes no No *NO*
57. My brother/sister pays attention to what I am saying.   *YES* Yes yes no No *NO*
58. When I really need to talk with my father, he is willing to listen.   *YES* Yes yes no No *NO*
59. I am troubled by headaches.   *YES* Yes yes no No *NO*
60. I worry a great deal about my family.   *YES* Yes yes no No *NO*
61. My mother pays attention to what I am saying.   *YES* Yes yes no No *NO*
62. My family members stand up for each other to outsiders.   *YES* Yes yes no No *NO*
63. I am bothered by nervousness, feeling fidgety or tense.   *YES* Yes yes no No *NO*
64. My father pays attention to what I am saying.   *YES* Yes yes no No *NO*
65. I have recently lost or gained weight.   *YES* Yes yes no No *NO*
66. When I really need to talk with my brother/sister, s/he is willing to listen.   *YES* Yes yes no No *NO*

6

A Measure of Denial in Coronary Clients: The Robinson Self-Appraisal Inventory

Karen R. Robinson

This chapter discusses the Robinson Self-Appraisal Inventory—Form D (RSAI-Form D), a measure of denial in persons with coronary heart disease.

PURPOSE

The purpose of this chapter is to present approaches used to refine and test the Robinson Self-Appraisal Inventory—Form D (RSAI-Form D) to measure denial in coronary clients. The use of denial by coronary clients is described extensively in the literature. However, little attention has been given to measuring it. In addition, clues that coronary clients are using denial may not be recognized through personal interviews or traditional assessment methods. Therefore, the Robinson Self-Appraisal Inventory (*RSAI*), a self-report assessment instrument was designed to identify denial in persons with coronary heart disease, quantify it, and aid in its further study (Robinson, 1994). It could also assist health care professionals to plan interventions to deal with denial.

CONCEPTUAL BASIS OF THE ROBINSON SELF-APPRAISAL INVENTORY

Denial in Coronary Heart Disease

Coronary heart disease, and the experiences associated with it, precipitate many sudden changes that severely disrupt the balance of psychosocial and environmental factors in an individual's life. Those who experience these changes use various resources, such as denial, in an attempt to cope with the anxiety caused by the various types of threatened or real losses associated with the myocardial infarction (Baas, Curl, Hertz, & Robinson, 1994; Cassem & Hackett, 1971; Fowers, 1992; Ketterer, et al., 1998; Lawrence & Lawrence, 1987/1988; Levine, Rudy, & Kerns, 1994; Robinson, 1988, 1990, 1993, 1994; Wielgosz, Nolan, Earp, Biro, & Wielgosz, 1988).

Denial is the ability of an individual to mentally ignore or push from consciousness the reality of the situation at hand. It is one of the first adaptive behaviors or mechanisms that a client uses during the stress-producing event of an acute episode of chest pain (Hackett & Cassem, 1982). For coronary clients, it is not difficult to use denial as a form of coping because once the pain has been alleviated and the client is comfortable, there are no other symptoms. The individual may rationalize or deny that anything significant has occurred. The ability to temporarily deny the meaning of an illness reduces the concomitant stress and anxiety caused by the loss and may be one factor that enhances the survival rate during the initial infarction period (Hackett, Cassem, & Wishnie, 1968). However, prolonged denial might cause the individual to ignore necessary activity restrictions, refuse to appreciate the significance of the illness, or fail to take prescribed medications needed to recover (Douglas & Druss, 1987; Fields, 1989).

Given that a myocardial infarction results in numerous real and threatened losses, and all loss, whether real, threatened, or perceived, produces a grief response, with denial, shock, and disbelief being the initial response (Engel, 1962), it becomes necessary to work through the grief process. However, this process should not be prolonged, as movement from denial to the next phase of the grief process might have a long-range effect on one's ability to work through the losses and changes in lifestyle caused by having coronary problems. Because denial does not represent a single, easily understood phenomenon, it is difficult to determine if it is adaptive or maladaptive (Owen, 1987).

Theoretical Perspective—Modeling and Role-Modeling

The Theory of Modeling and Role-Modeling, developed by Erickson, Tomlin, and Swain (1988), provided the explanatory framework for the development of the RSAI-Form D. This nursing theory maintains that the client's perception of the situation is based on a unique model of the world that is gradually and continually constructed. The client's behavior reflects the model and provides information about the level of psychosocial development attained and the available coping adaptive mechanisms.

An assumption in the Modeling and Role-Modeling theory is that all people have a drive toward maximum growth and development across the life span. This drive has at its core instinctive needs that motivate behavior. When needs are met repeatedly, development occurs. Objects that repeatedly meet needs take on significance for the individuals; thus, an attachment to the object occurs. Loss of the attachment results in the grief response (Lindemann, 1944). It is necessary to work through the grief process and reattach to a new object in order to contend fully with the stressors of everyday life.

The extent of loss a client experiences is directly related to the individual's emotional attachment to the lost object. Clients with coronary disease often have an attachment to their previous heart function, body image, or self-image. Whenever there is an event such as an acute episode of chest pain that threatens loss of this attachment object, a grief response occurs, with denial and shock the first stage of the process (Engel, 1962). When the individual is initially confronted with this sense of loss, denial may provide the necessary time to perceive an adequate alternative attachment object. Resolution of the loss and grief is obtained by needs being successfully met for the coronary client with an attachment occurring to the object meeting those needs (Erickson et al., 1988).

PROCEDURES FOR DEVELOPMENT

The RSAI has been under development for approximately 10 years. Earlier studies led to revisions and reconceptualizations (Robinson, 1982; 1988), which have resulted in Form D. The original (RSAI) was developed in 1982 (Robinson, 1982). Even though the Hackett-Cassem Denial Scale was available for measuring denial, there was a concern about the number of items on the scale regarding patients' personality traits and behaviors not related to their illness (e.g. risk taking) and the general use of denial as a defensive trait. An additional weakness of this measurement was that the nature of several questions in the scale required the interviewer to make inferences when rating denial behavioral characteristics of the participant; it was not a paper–and–pencil self-report (Hackett & Cassem, 1974). Rather than measuring traits, the RSAI directly focuses on the patients' present reactions to their illness and it is designed as a paper–and–pencil, self-administered instrument.

An attempt was made to identify the essence of the construct of denial by conducting a concept analysis. Then the Hackett-Cassem Denial Scale was studied to determine which of the 31 interview questions generated appropriate content related to denial in coronary clients. Thirteen of the questions were selected and rewritten so that participants could respond to each of them on a four-point Likert-type scale (Robinson, 1982). For example, in the Hackett-Cassem Scale, the interviewer responds *yes* or *no* to item 8, which reads, "Did the client admit a fear of death at any time?" The statement was rewritten to read, "I have a concern about death," with possible responses ranging from 1 = strongly agree to 4 = strongly disagree. Additional items were added to measure the various aspects of the construct that had been identified in concept analysis. Cardiovascular and psychiatric clinical nurse specialists and critical care nurse experts judged the newly developed instrument's content validity.

Three studies (Robinson, 1982, 1988, 1994) have been conducted that have resulted in the further development and evolution of the RSAI-Form D. These studies are described in the reliability and validity section of this chapter in Table 6.1.

DESCRIPTION

The RSAI–Form D consists of 20 statements, with responses entered on a five-point Likert-type scale (see Appendix). Participants are instructed to give their first reaction to how they feel about each statement (e.g., " I don't spend much time thinking about the possibility that the chest pain may return," "I don't really believe that there is anything wrong with my heart," "At present my main worry is my health"). Participants respond to each statement by selecting one of the following: (1) *strongly agree*, (2) *agree* (3) *uncertain*, (4) *disagree*, or (5) *strongly disagree*.

ADMINISTRATION AND SCORING

The RSAI- Form D is designed to be self-administered and to be given on an individual basis. It requires five to ten minutes to administer to those individuals who have average or above average reading ability. An individual is able to complete it without the assistance of others. The original instrument, the RSAI, was assessed for reading level using the computer program *RightWriter* (1986) by Shirley Ziegler, PhD, RN, Professor, Texas Woman's University. The obtained readability index of 3.17 indicated that readers needed a third-grade level of education to understand the RSAI items.

Half of the items (e.g., "I am seriously ill") are worded in such a manner that a rating of (5) indicates a high level of denial, while the other half of the items (e.g., "I don't really believe that there is anything wrong with my heart") are worded so that a high rating indicates low denial. The score for each item on which a high rating indicates high denial is the same as the response number circled for that item on the test form (items 1, 4, 5, 10, 11, 14, 15, 16, 18, and 20). For items on which a high rating indicates low denial, the item scores are reversed; that is, responses numbered 1, 2, 3, 4, or 5, are scored 5, 4, 3, 2, and 1, respectively. The denial items for which the scoring is reversed on the inventory are 2, 3, 6, 7, 8, 9, 12, 13, 17, and 19.

To obtain scores for the RSAI-Form D, the scores for the 20 items that make up the inventory are added, taking into consideration the 10 scores that are reversed. Scores for the RSAI-Form D can range from a minimum score of 20 to a maximum score of 100.

RELIABILITY AND VALIDITY EVIDENCE

Table 6.1 summarizes the studies that have been done to assess the psychometric properties of the RSAI.

CONCLUSIONS AND RECOMMENDATIONS

The purpose of the most recent study was to refine and test the RSAI-Form D, a scale designed to measure denial in actual or potential myocardial infarction clients (Robinson, 1994). Although the findings from this study are tentative, given the nature of this convenience sample and the utilization of an exploratory research design, preliminary evidence was obtained that the RSAI-Form D is a reliable and valid research instrument.

Factor analysis indicated that the 20–item RSAI-Form D probably is a multidimensional measure; however, a larger sample is needed with the addition of items to the scale to make the final determination. Four aspects of denial were extracted, thus providing supportive evidence to the health care professional that using single specific or global criteria does not provide sufficient data for assessing denial. Some individuals may use one type of denial, whereas others may use another type. Each type of denial has its own purpose for the person and could be denial of secondary consequences, denial of illness and treatment, denial of anxiety, or denial of impact. Therefore, it is beneficial for the health care professional to observe and listen closely to clients to understand their perspective as well as determine the type of denial that is being utilized (Robinson, 1994).

Based on the findings of the past studies, which aided in the development of the RSAI-Form D, the following recommendations for future studies are made:

1. A qualitative study needs to be conducted to document and interpret, as fully as possible, the first stage of the grief process—denial—from the frame of reference of the participants involved. This would allow delineation and specification of the construct of denial to be as complete as possible so that representative items could be integrated into the RSAI–Form D.

TABLE 6.1 Reliability and Validity Evidence of the RSAI-Form D

Study citation	Sample and characteristics	Reliability evidence	Validity evidence
Robinson, K. R. (1982). *Denial and anxiety in second day myocardial infarction patients.* Unpublished master's thesis, Texas Woman's University, Denton, TX.	*Sample Size:* 30 *Characteristics:* Male myocardial infarction patients with a mean age of 48 years. None of the participants had experienced a previous myocardial infarction.	*Internal Consistency:* coefficient alpha = 0.65 indicating a low level of homogeneity among the 20 items of the RSAI.	*Construct Validity:* A relationship between denial and state anxiety should exist (Bigos, 1981; Hackett, Cassem, & Wishnie, 1968). Even though the hypothesis was rejected at the .05 level ($p = .07$), the relationship between denial and state anxiety variables was in the predicted direction in that as denial levels increased, state anxiety levels decreased. The mean state anxiety score was 37.17 and the mean denial score was 45.
Robinson, K. R. (1988). Denial and anxiety in second day myocardial infarction patients. In C. F. Waltz & O. L. Strickland (Eds.), *Measurement of Nursing Outcomes* (Vol. 1) (pp. 47—60). New York: Springer.	*Sample Size:* 26 *Characteristics:* The sample consisted of 19 men and 7 women with recent myocardial infarctions. Mean age was 57 years. One participant had experienced a previous myocardial infarction.	*Internal Consistency:* Coefficient alpha = 0.41. Inter-item correlations ranged from 0.24 to 0.74. When the 5 items with a variance greater than 1.046 were removed from the scale, the alpha value increased to 0.62	*Construct Validity:* Findings revealed second day post myocardial infarction patients with higher denial scores had lower state anxiety scores when trait anxiety was controlled; this relationship was statistically significant ($p = .0001$). The mean state anxiety score was 35.9 and the mean denial score was 47.5.
Robinson, K.R. (1994). Developing a scale to measure denial levels of clients with actual or potential myocardial	*Sample Size:* 130 *Characteristics:* The sample consisted of 108 men and 22 women hospitalized with actual	*Internal Consistency:* Coefficient alpha = 0.80 for both the second and fourth day scores. Form D was determined to be	*Factor Analysis:* Construct validity was assessed by determining whether the items in the RSAI-Form D measured a unidimensional construct of denial and, consequently, whether the RSAI-Form D was a unidimensional scale. Factor analysis indicated that the

TABLE 6.1 (*continued*)

Study citation	Sample and characteristics	Reliability evidence	Validity evidence
infarctions. *Heart & Lung: The Journal of Critical Care, 23*(1), 36–44.	or potential myocardial infarction. Average age was 60.9 years.	internally consistent. Item-total analysis revealed the reliability of the overall scale could not be dramatically improved by deleting an item.	RSAI-Form D probably is a multidimensional measurement instrument. However, results of the Day 2 and Day 4 oblique rotations revealed that some items did not load on the same factor, so Day 2 and Day 4 factors were identified and named according to the definition of the items. The four Day 2 factors were identified as follows: Factor 1—"Denial of secondary consequences," Factor 2—"Denial of illness and treatment," Factor 3—"Denial of anxiety," and Factor 4—"Denial of impact." The Day 4 factors were identified as follows: Factor 1—"Developing an awareness of illness and treatment," Factor 2—"Developing an awareness of illness and secondary consequences," Factor 3—"Developing an awareness of anxiety," and Factor 4—"Developing an awareness of impact" (Robinson, 1994). The factors are similar to aspects of denial reported in the literature, thus providing some support for content and construct validity of the RSAI-Form D (Hackett et al., 1968; Havik & Maeland, 1986; Weisman, 1972).
			Day 2 RSAI-Form D scores ranged from 30 to 82 with an average score of 55.07, whereas the Day 4 scores for the group ranged from 27 to 74 with a mean score of 51.19. Statistical results revealed a significant decrease in mean scores from the second to the fourth hospitalized day.

2. Follow-up studies should be conducted with a further refined and expanded version of the RSAI-Form D.
3. Further factor analytic studies need to be conducted with large ethnically and racially diverse samples. According to Kerlinger (1986), factor analytic studies need to be replicated with as large a sample as possible. "The 'reality' of factors is much more compelling if found in two or three different and large samples" (p. 593).

In conclusion, there is evidence that supports the reliability and validity of the RSAI-Form D. However, further psychometric work is needed to further enhance its performance as a measure of denial in coronary heart disease clients.

REFERENCES

Baas, L. S., Curl, E. D., Hertz, J. E., & Robinson, K. R. (1994). Innovative approaches to theory based measurement: Modeling and role modeling research. In P. L. Chinn (Ed.), *Advances in methods of inquiry for nursing,* (pp. 147–159). Gaithersburg, MD: Aspen.

Bigos, K. M. (1981). Behavioral adaptation during the acute phase of a myocardial infarction. *Western Journal of Nursing Research, 3,* 150–167.

Cassem, N. H., & Hackett, T. P. (1971). Psychiatric consultation in a coronary care unit. *Annals of Internal Medicine, 75,* 9–14.

Douglas, C. J., & Druss, R. G. (1987). Denial of illness: A reappraisal. *General Hospital Psychiatry, 9,* 53–57.

Engel, G. L. (1962*). Psychological development in health and disease.* Philadelphia: Saunders.

Erickson, H. C., Tomlin, E. M., & Swain, M. A. (1988). *Modeling and role-modeling: A theory and paradigm for nursing.* Lexington, SC: Pine Press of Lexington.

Fields, K. B. (1989). Myocardial infarction and denial. *Journal of Family Practice, 28,* 157–161.

Fowers, B. J. (1992). The cardiac denial of impact scale: A brief, self-report research measure. *Journal of Psychosomatic Research, 36,* 469–475.

Hackett, T. P., & Cassem, N. H. (1974). Development of a quantitative rating scale to assess denial. *Journal of Psychosomatic Research, 18,* 93–100.

Hackett, T. P., & Cassem, N. H. (1982). Coping with cardiac disease. *Advanced Cardiology, 31,* 212–217.

Hackett, T. P., Cassem, N. H., & Wishnie, H. A. (1968). The coronary care unit: An appraisal of its psychological hazards. *New England Journal of Medicine, 279,* 1365–1370.

Havik, O. E., & Maeland, J. G. (1986). Dimensions of verbal denial in myocardial infarction. *Scandinavian Journal of Psychology, 27,* 326–339.

Kerlinger, F. N. (1986). *Foundations of behavioral research* (3rd ed.). New York: Holt, Rinehart, and Winston.

Ketterer, M. W., Huffman, J., Lumley, M. A., Wassef, S., Gray, L., Kenyon, L., Kraft, P., Brymer, J., Rhoads, K., Lovallo, W. R., & Goldberg, A. D. (1998). Five-year follow-up for adverse outcomes in males with at least minimally positive angiograms: Importance of "denial" in assessing psychosocial risk factors. *Journal of Psychosomatic Research, 44,* 241–250.

Lawrence, S. A., & Lawrence, R. M. (1987/1988). Helping patients to cope with the stress of myocardial infarction. *Nursing Forum, 23*(3), 92–100.

Levine, J., Rudy, T., & Kerns, R. (1994). A two factor model of denial of illness: A confirmatory factor analysis. *Journal of Psychosomatic Research, 38,* 99–110.

Lindemann, E. (1944). Symptomatology and management of acute grief. *American Journal of Psychiatry, 101,* 141–148.

Owen, P. M. (1987). Recovery from myocardial infarction: A review of psychosocial determinants. *Journal of Cardiovascular Nursing, 2,* 75–85.

Robinson, K. R. (1982). *Denial and anxiety in second day myocardial infarction patients.* Unpublished master's thesis, Texas Woman's University, Denton, TX.

Robinson, K. R. (1988). Denial and anxiety in second day myocardial infarction patients. In C. F. Waltz & O. L. Strickland (Eds.), *Measurement of nursing outcomes: Vol. 1: Client outcome* (pp. 47–60). New York: Springer Publishing Co.

Robinson, K. R. (1990). Denial in myocardial infarction patients. *Critical Care Nurse, 10*(5), 138–145.

Robinson, K. R. (1993). Denial: An adaptive response. *Dimensions of Critical Care Nursing, 12*(2), 102–106.

Robinson, K. R. (1994). Developing a scale to measure denial levels of clients with actual or potential myocardial infarctions. *Heart & Lung: Journal of Critical Care, 23*(1), 36–44.

Weisman, A. D. (1972). *On dying and denying: A psychiatric study of terminality.* New York: Behavioral Publications.

Wielgosz, A. T., Nolan, R. P., Earp, J. A., Biro, E., & Wielgosz, M. B. (1988). Reasons for patients' delay in response to symptoms of acute myocardial infarction. *Canadian Medical Association Journal, 139,* 853–857.

APPENDIX: ROBINSON SELF-APPRAISAL INVENTORY-FORM D (RSAI-FORM D)

Directions: A number of statements which people have used to describe how they feel are given below. Please carefully read each statement. Circle the number of the answer which best indicates how you feel about these statements. Please give your *first reaction* to the statement. There are no right or wrong answers.

Please answer according to the following key:

1. STRONGLY AGREE
2. AGREE
3. UNCERTAIN
4. DISAGREE
5. STRONGLY DISAGREE

1. I am seriously ill.	1 2 3 4 5
2. I don't spend much time thinking about the possibility that the chest pain may return.	1 2 3 4 5
3. I feel that my doctor has placed too many restrictions on me.	1 2 3 4 5
4. I have a concern about death.	1 2 3 4 5
5. I worry that I will be an invalid.	1 2 3 4 5
6. Since I feel fine, I think that my doctor should send me home.	1 2 3 4 5
7. At the present time, I don't feel anxious.	1 2 3 4 5
8. I try to forget everything about heart disease.	1 2 3 4 5
9. The less time that I think about my illness, the better.	1 2 3 4 5
10. I am afraid that the chest pain will come back.	1 2 3 4 5
11. I wish that the doctors and nurses would tell me more often that I am doing well.	1 2 3 4 5
12. I don't really believe that there is anything wrong with my heart.	1 2 3 4 5
13. The proverb, "let sleeping dogs lie," reflects my present feelings.	1 2 3 4 5
14. I feel the need to learn more about heart disease.	1 2 3 4 5
15. At present my heart is not strong enough for me to walk up a flight of stairs.	1 2 3 4 5
16. At present my main worry is my health.	1 2 3 4 5
17. It doesn't do me any good to worry about my heart.	1 2 3 4 5
18. I am more worried about my health than my doctor is.	1 2 3 4 5
19. My family is more worried about my health than I am.	1 2 3 4 5
20. I feel that I need to follow my doctor's instructions.	1 2 3 4 5

©Karen Robinson, PhD, RN, Department of Veterans Affairs Medical Center, 2101 Elm Street, Fargo, North Dakota 58102.

7

Measuring Stress After Acute Myocardial Infarction: The Stress of Discharge Assessment Tool, Version Two (SDAT-2)

Jean C. Toth

This chapter presents the Stress of Discharge Assessment Tool, Version Two (SDAT-2), a measure of the impact of stressors common to acute myocardial infarction (AMI) patients at hospital discharge and in the early recovery period at home.

PURPOSE

The purpose of the Stress of Discharge Assessment Tool, Version Two (SDAT-2), is to measure the impact of stressors common to acute myocardial infarction (AMI) patients at hospital discharge and during early recovery at home. These stressors include recovery from the illness, family difficulties, and the anticipation of or actual problems experienced by AMI patients.

CONCEPTUAL BASIS OF THE STRESS OF DISCHARGE ASSESSMENT TOOL

The Psychophysiologic/Spiritual Stress Model, developed by Toth (1980, 1988, 1992), illustrates the interplay of multiple physiological, psychological, environmental, sociocultural, and spiritual stressors on affective and physiologic behavior (see Figure 7.1). Examples of physiological stressors include the immediate effects of myocardial tissue damage/death and angina, found to be present in 50% of patients in the two weeks following AMI (Toth, 1987a). Psychological stressors include anxiety, anger (Newton & Froelicher, 1995), depression, disappointment over the illness, and

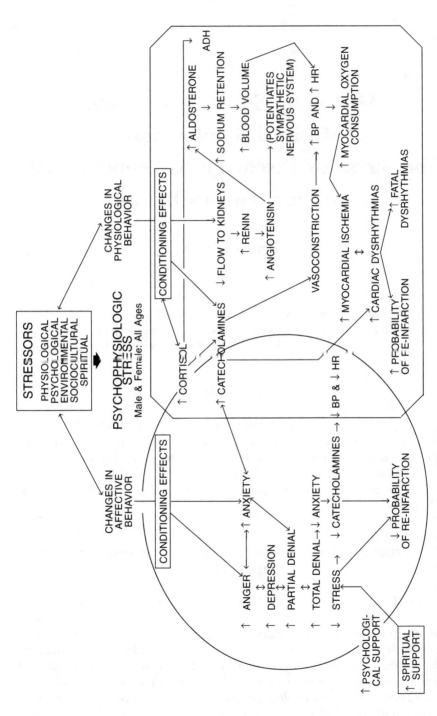

FIGURE 7.1 Psychophysiologic Stress Model.

worry about another MI (Toth, 1987a). Environmental stressors for AMI patients are pollution and intense heat or cold (McCance & Huether, 1998).

Sociocultural stressors include inability to perform customary roles as spouse, parent, homemaker, or employee (Speedling, 1982), and that the partner (or important person) worries too much about them (also a psychological stressor) (Toth 1987a, 1992). Similarly, research results indicate that of sexually active AMI patients, 31.3% reported that after their doctor says it is all right for them to resume sexual activities, their partner would be worried about that (Toth, 1987a).

Although a common spiritual stressor with AMI patients is the feeling that somehow God let them down, research using this Model shows that their spiritual thinking (the meaning of life or religious background) consistently helped them to feel better (Toth, 1992). This was also true of their partners (Toth, 1999). In addition, the Model also illustrates how the presence of these multiple stressors increases the likelihood of complications and relapse following AMI. Interestingly, research using the Model has also shown that stress at hospital discharge affects men and women equally (Toth, 1993), and that the magnitude of stress and type of stressors in younger and old AMI patients are the same (Toth, 1987a, 1988).

Stress, a nonspecific response of the body to any demand made upon it (Selye, 1980; McCance & Huether, 1998), occurs in response to the number and magnitude of stressors, modified by what Selye described as conditioning effects (individual differences). Changes in affective behavior lead to changes in physiological behavior and conversely, also. The basic assumption underlying this Model is that stress is not desirable during early recovery following AMI.

PROCEDURES FOR DEVELOPMENT

The SDAT has two versions—the SDAT-1 and the SDAT-2. Both have 60 items. The SDAT-2 is currently in use.

The SDAT-1

Content for the initial version of the SDAT was determined through a review of the literature, clinical experience, interviews with former AMI patients and their families, and through an eight-member panel of experts in cardiovascular clinical nursing practice and education, and educational testing. The panel was also used for content validation.

Construct validity was evaluated by the concurrent administration of the Anxiety-Depression (A-D) Scale for Medically Ill Patients (Sgroi, Holland, & Solkoff, 1970). The A-D Scale contains anxiety (15 items) and depression (13 items) subscales. Pearson product-moment correlations between scores on the SDAT and the Anxiety Subscale [$r(104)$ = .18, p = .03] and the Depression Subscale [$r(104)$ = .34, $p < .001$] were statistically significant but low to moderately low in magnitude. Even so, these findings lend some evidence for the validity of the constructs of anxiety (4 items) and depression (5 items) of the SDAT. Also, as the A-D Scale measures only anxiety and depression, some support exists for the discriminant validity of the SDAT for the remaining items (Toth, 1988).

Items for the SDAT were written on an eighth grade literacy level. No differences were found in scores between subjects who were able to read and those to whom the SDAT was read [$t(102) > .05$, NS; $t(88)$ = .38, p = .71, NS on pretest; $t(88)$ = .63, p = .53, NS on posttest]. Approximately 1/3 of the 1987a study subjects of Toth and 12.2% of the 1992 sample were functionally illiterate; that is, were unable to read or unable to understand what they read.

The SDAT-2

Item analysis from the SDAT-1 was used to measure the contribution of individual items to the total score and to guide revisions of the SDAT. Any items with an item to total correlation of < .20 were revised. These revisions were minor and included the rewording of items to improve clarity and to reflect the magnitude of stress AMI patients experience whether answering the tool at hospital discharge or during recovery at home. The revisions were reviewed by panel members and resulted in the SDAT-2.

DESCRIPTION OF THE SDAT-2

The SDAT-2 is a 60–item self-report Likert scale questionnaire. It has two parts. Part A has 46 items that measure stressors common to most AMI patients. There are five possible responses to each of the items: SA = *strongly agree*, A = *agree*, U = *uncertain*, D = *disagree*, SD = *strongly disagree*. Part B contains 14 items that measure stressors that may not be common to all AMI patients, so an additional response is added, or NA = does not apply to me.

Table 7.1 shows content areas. Items measure how these patients are feeling at the time of taking the test; they are not intended to measure knowledge.

ADMINISTRATION AND SCORING

The SDAT-2 is a paper-and-pencil questionnaire that takes approximately 15 minutes to answer. (See Appendix). It measures stress that AMI pa-

TABLE 7.1 Content Areas of the SDAT–2

Content area*	Number of items
A. Feelings toward self	
1. Control	5
2. Depression	5
3. Perceived knowledge	5
4. Anxiety	4
5. Denial	3
6. Ready to go home	3
7. Severity of illness	2
8. Spirituality	1
	(28)
B. Feelings towards others	
1. Social support	7
2. Communication	5
3. Responsibility to others	1
	(13)
C. Anticipation of problems	
1. Home related	13
2. Work (financial) related	6
	(19)

*N=60 items.

tients experience at hospital discharge (zero to 48 hours prior to going home) and/or during early recovery at home (12 to 14 days after hospital discharge). It can be read by the patient or to the patient by the researcher.

Scores range from one to five points for each item. Total scores range from 60 to 300 points with a high score indicating high stress.

Points are assigned in the following way: SA = 1, A = 2, U = 3, D = 4, SD or NA = 1. Scores on 21 of the 60 items are recoded (1 = 5, 2 = 4, 3 = 3, 4 = 2, 5 = 1) prior to the summation of total scores. The following items are recoded: 2, 8, 10, 16, 17, 19, 25, 27, 29, 31, 34, 43, 45, 48, 51, 52, 54, 55, 56, and 59 (Toth 1987b).

RELIABILITY AND VALIDITY EVIDENCE

Evidence for the reliability and validity of the SDAT has been shown in several studies, as indicated in Table 7.2.

TABLE 7.2 Reliability and Validity of the SDAT

Study citation	Sample and characteristics	Reliability evidence	Validity evidence
Toth, J. C. (1988). Measuring the stressful experience of hospital discharge following acute myocardial infarction. In C. F. Waltz, & O. L. Strickland (Eds.). *Measurement of Nursing Outcomes, Vol. One* (pp. 3–23). New York: Springer.	*Sample:* N = 104. *Characteristics:* Age 38–86, M = 63.6 years, Education 1–22 M = 12.0 years, Race 77.9% white (n = 81), Black 22.1% (n = 23); Gender, male 76% (n = 79), female 24% (n = 25). *Setting:* 3 acute care hospitals. *Diagnosis:* AMI. *Purpose:* to develop an instrument to measure the stress AMI patients experience at hospital discharge and to identify variables that may be predictors of this stress.	*Internal consistency reliability:* r = .85 *Item-to-total correlations* for the 60 items that met criterion of >.15 were 53 items (88.3%).	*Content validity:* Review of the literature, content validation by a panel of experts. *Criterion-related validity:* Concurrent validity with Anxiety-Depression Scale for Medically Ill Patients (Sgroi, Holland, & Solkoff, 1970); r(104) = .18 on anxiety and r(104) = .34 on depression.
Toth, J. C. (1986). Unpublished data.	*Sample:* N = 20. *Characteristics:* Mean Age = 53.7 years, Mean Education = 14.6 years, Race = 100% White, Gender = male 80%, female 20%. *Setting:* Acute care hospital. *Diagnosis:* AMI. *Purpose of Pilot Study:* To evaluate the 2nd version of the SDAT.	Randomly assigned to two groups. One group answered SDAT-1, other SDAT-2. *Internal consistency:* SDAT-1 was r = .73, SDAT-2 was r = .84. *Item-to-total correlations:* >.20, n = 49 (81.7%) of items.	*Criterion related validity:* Concurrent validity of SDAT-1 with SDAT-2 scores; also met test for homogeneity of variance (F = 2.2, p > .05, NS).

TABLE 7.2 (continued)

Study citation	Sample and characteristics	Reliability evidence	Validity evidence
Toth, J. C. (1987a). Stressors affecting older and younger acute myocardial infarction patients at hospital discharge. *Dimensions in Critical Care Nursing, 6*(3), 147–157.	*Sample:N* = 104. (Re-analysis of data from 1988 study.) *Characteristics:* Age 38–86, *M* = 63.6 years; Education 1–22, Mean = 12.0 years, Race 77.9% White (*n* = 81), black 22.1% (*n* = 23); Gender, male 76% (*n* = 79), female 24% (*n* = 25). *Setting:* Three acute care hospitals. *Diagnosis:* AMI. *Purpose:* to compare stressors affecting older AMI patients to stressors affecting younger AMI patients at hospital discharge.	*Internal consistency reliability: r* = .85 (re-analysis of data)	*Construct validity:* The 3 most stressful items were the *same* for both older (*n* = 48) and younger (*n* = 56) AMI patients: Content of these items were disappointment (item 10), partner worries too much (item 48), and disbelief (item 16). *Construct Validity:* Supported hypothesis that stress is not age specific after AMI [*t*(102) = .03, p.98, NS]; supported hypothesis that the perception of the partners' worries about resumption of sexual activities is also not age specific [chi sq.(4) = 6.1, p.19, NS].
Toth, J. C. (1992). Faith in recovery: Spiritual support after an acute MI. *Journal of Christian Nursing, 9*(4), 28–31.	*Sample: N* = 90. *Characteristics:* Mean Age = 55.5 years, Education Mean = 14.2 years, Race 93.3% White, Black 4.4%, other 3.3%; Gender, male 80%, female 20%.	*Internal consistency reliability:* Pretest .85, posttest .89. *Item-to-total correlations:* Pretest with 50 items (83.3%) were >.20; posttest 53 items (88.3%) were >.20.	*Construct validity:* Supported by theory since subjects who reported more spiritual support at home had less stress at home [*r*(90) = −.28,p = .003] and spiritual support was stable over time [*r*(90) = .70, *p* = .001].

TABLE 7.2 *(continued)*

Study citation	Sample and characteristics	Reliability evidence	Validity evidence
	Setting: Pretests at an acute care hospital & posttests in subjects homes. *Diagnosis:* AMI. *Purpose:* to compare the spiritual support AMI patients experience at hospital discharge to spiritual support at home.		
Toth, J. C. (1993). Is stress at hospital discharge after acute myocardial infarction greater in women than in men? *American Journal of Critical Care, 2*(1),35–40.	*Sample: N* = 104. Re-analysis of data from two combined studies (1988 & 1992). *Characteristics:* Age 38–82, *M* = 62.8 years; Education 3–19, *M* = 12.7 years; Race 92.6% White, black 7.4%, other 3.3%; Gender; male 77.1% (*n* = 182), female 22.9% (*n* = 54). *Setting:* Four acute care hospitals. *Diagnosis:* AMI. *Purpose:* To compare the level of stress experienced by women and men at hospital discharge after AMI.	*Internal consistency reliability:* Males .85, females .83.	*Construct Validity:* Supported hypothesis that stress at hospital discharge following AMI is not gender specific. [$t(234)$ = .4, $p > .05$, NS].

TABLE 7.2 (continued)

Study citation	Sample and characteristics	Reliability evidence	Validity evidence
Toth, J. C. (1999). Faith in God: Help for partners in pain. *Journal of Christian Nursing, 16*(2), 19–21.*	*Sample:* N = 23. *Characteristics:* Age 45–84 years; Education 12 years (60.9%) < 12 years (29.1%); Gender 100% women. *Setting:* Government hospital & patients' homes. *Diagnosis:* Partners of patients with coronary artery disease: Coronary by-pass graft surgery (CABG) (43.5%), AMI (30.5%) & AMI &/or angioplasty (PTCA) (13.0%). *Purpose:* To measure the reliability of the Partner Stress Assessment Tool (PSAT) developed from the SDAT-2 and to identify stressors of partners of AMI patients surrounding hospital discharge of the patients.	*Internal consistency reliability:* 0.93	*Content validity:* Panel of experts, review of the literature, interviews of partners of AMI, CABG, & PTCA patients, & clinical experience. *Construct validity:* Spiritual support of partners reduces their stress: (91.3% said their spirituality helped them (item 24) , and 95.7% found strength in God (item 45) and that prayer was an important source of comfort to them (item 44).

*Data collected and shared by Lois Camberg, PhD and Pat Woods, RN, MS, Veterans Affairs Medical Center, Roxbury, Mass.

CONCLUSIONS AND RECOMMENDATIONS

The Stress of Discharge Assessment Tool (SDAT) has been found to be a consistently reliable measure of the magnitude of stress that AMI patients experience at hospital discharge. Its validity is supported through the literature and research findings related to continued development of the Psychophysiologic/Spiritual Stress Model. This Model was specifically expanded through data collected using the SDAT to include the positive effect of reduction in stress provided by a person's spirituality. In AMI patients, who have been so acutely ill, this finding on spirituality is indeed good news to the patients, their families, and nurses who now have re-search to support the need of AMI patients for spiritual care. The series of studies that have used the SDAT indicates that the theoretical con-struct of spiritual support reduces stress, and that stress following AMI at hospital discharge is neither gender nor age related.

The Partner Stress Assessment Tool (PSAT) has been developed from the SDAT to measure the stress of partners of persons who have had an AMI. The items are similar to those on the SDAT, and the PSAT has undergone initial psychometric assessment.

More testing needs to be done with the SDAT to evaluate its ability to measure the effect of intervention programs for patients and their part-ners. In addition, the psychometric properties of the SDAT-2 would be enhanced by its use and assessment in more ethnically and racially di-verse samples. More evidence of the reliability and validity of the SDAT-2 is likely to become available, as requests for copies of the SDAT-2 have been made by nurse and non-nurse researchers, graduate nursing stu-dents, nursing educators, and hospital chaplains. These requests have come from individuals in the USA and in foreign countries.

Requests for a copy of the PSAT may be made by writing to Dr. Jean C. Toth, RN, School of Nursing, The Catholic University of America, Washington, DC 20064 (toth@cua.edu).

REFERENCES

McCance, K. L., & Huether, S. E. (1998). *Pathophysiology: The biologic basis for disease in adults and children* (3rd ed). St. Louis: Mosby.

Newton, K. M., & Froelicher, E. S. S. (1995). Coronary heart disease risk factors. In S. L. Woods, E. S. S. Froelicher, C. J. Halpenny & S. U. Motzer (Eds.), *Cardiac nursing* (3rd ed.),(pp. 200–211). Philadelphia, PA: J. B. Lippincott.

Selye, H. (1980). Stress and a holistic view of health for the nursing pro-fession. In K. E. Claus, & J. T. Bailey (Eds.). *Living with stress and promoting well-being*. St. Louis: Mosby.

Sgroi, S. M., Holland, J. C. B., & Solkoff, N. (1970). *Development of an Anxiety-Depression Scale for use with medically ill patients* (Mimeograph). New York: Department of Psychiatry, School of Medicine, State University of New York at Buffalo.

Speedling, E. J. (1982). *Heart attack: The family response at home and in the hospital.* New York: Tavistock.

Toth, J. C. (1980). Effect of structured preparation for transfer on patient anxiety on leaving coronary care unit. *Nursing Research, 29,* 28–34.

Toth, J. C. (1986). Unpublished data. School of Nursing, The Catholic University of America, Washington, DC.

Toth, J. C. (1987a). Stressors affecting older and younger acute myocardial infarction patients at hospital discharge. *Dimensions in Critical Care Nursing, 6*(3), 147–157.

Toth, J. C. (1987b). *The Stress of Discharge Assessment Tool (SDAT) following acute myocardial infarction, Version Two.* Circulated manuscript.

Toth, J. C. (1988). Measuring the stressful experience of hospital discharge following acute myocardial infarction. In C. F. Waltz & O. L. Strickland (Eds.), *Measurement of nursing outcomes: Vol. 1: Measuring client outcomes* (pp. 3–23). New York: Springer Publishing Co.

Toth, J. C. (1992). Faith in recovery: Spiritual support after an acute MI. *Journal of Christian Nursing, 9*(4), 28–31.

Toth, J. C. (1993). Is stress at hospital discharge after acute myocardial infarction greater in women than in men? *American Journal of Critical Care, 2*(1), 35–40.

Toth, J. C. (1999). Faith in God: Help for partners in pain. *Journal of Christian Nursing, 16*(2), 19–21.

APPENDIX: PATIENT SURVEY SDAT   Code No. _____ (1-4)

Version Two©   Card No. _____ (5)

Part A

Directions: All of the statements in this Part (1 through 46) refer to how you are feeling now. There are five possible responses to each of the statements. They are:

> SA = Strongly Agree
> A = Agree
> U = Uncertain
> D = Disagree
> SD = Strongly Disagree

For each statement, circle the letter(s) that best describes your feeling.

1. I was glad to learn that I was going home from the hospital.   SA A U D SD
2. I feel more nervous today than I usually do.   SA A U D SD
3. When I found out I was going home from the hospital it made me feel that my health was getting better.   SA A U D SD
   SA A U D SD
4. I am sure that I had a heart attack.   SA A U D SD
5. I slept well last night.   SA A U D SD
6. I was not very sick when I first got to the hospital.   SA A U D SD
7. My spiritual thinking (the meaning of life or religious background) has helped me to feel better about myself.   SA A U D SD
8. I felt a little worried when I found out that I was about to leave the hospital.   SA A U D SD
9. My appetite is good today.   SA A U D SD
10. I feel disappointed that I got sick.   SA A U D SD
11. When I found out I was going home from the hospital I felt ready to go.   SA A U D SD
12. I have at least one person that I feel I can talk to about myself or my problems.   SA A U D SD
13. I feel it is all right to ask the doctors or the nurses questions I have about my illness.   SA A U D SD
14. I am able to tell the difference between heart pain (angina) and ordinary aches and pains.   SA A U D SD
15. I have asked my doctor or nurse questions about my illness since I have been here.   SA A U D SD
16. I find it hard to believe that this illness happened to me.   SA A U D SD

Please go to the next page

Key: SA = Strongly Agree
A = Agree
U = Uncertain
D = Disagree
SD = Strongly Disagree

17. I was having financial problems before I got sick.   SA A U D SD
18. I understand what physical activities I can do.   SA A U D SD
19. I feel depressed today.   SA A U D SD
20. When I asked questions about my illness I   SA A U D SD
understood the answers the doctors gave me.
21. After my doctor says it is all right, I believe that my SA A U D SD
illness will not make much difference in my sexual
activities.
22. I know what specific conditions I should report to   SA A U D SD
my doctor or nurse, if they happen to me.
23. I understand what physical activities I should not   SA A U D SD
do.
24. When I asked questions about my Illness, I   SA A U D SD
understood the answers that the nurses gave me.
25. I feel tired today.   SA A U D SD
26. I plan to do things differently than before I got   SA A U D SD
sick.
27. Being in the hospital has resulted in a financial   SA A U D SD
problem for me.
28. I think it is all right to contact my doctor or nurse   SA A U D SD
if I have questions about my care.
29. Sometimes I worry if I will be able to stay calm.   SA A U D SD
30. I have one or more people who depend on me to   SA A U D SD
take care of them.
31. Sometimes I do not know what questions to ask my SA A U D SD
doctor or nurse about my illness.
32. Getting extremely upset about things is not good for SA A U D SD
me now.
33. I understand why I got sick.   SA A U D SD
34. I sometimes worry that I will not be able to take care SA A U D SD
of myself.
35. When I compare myself to other people with my   SA A U D SD
kind of illness, I think that mv progress in getting
well has been as good as theirs.
36. I will be able to make the changes in my everyday   SA A U D SD
living that my doctor or nurse has suggested.
37. I fell the same or better about myself now, than   SA A U D SD
before I got sick.
38. I understand what foods I should not eat.   SA A U D SD

Please go to the next page

Key: SA = Strongly Agree
         A = Agree
         U = Uncertain
         D = Disagree
         SD = Strongly Disagree

39. Feeling weak is a normal reaction for people with my   SA A U D SD
    illness.
40. I know what to do if I get any heart pain (angina).   SA A U D SD
41. I know how to get in touch with my doctor or   SA A U D SD
    nurse.
42. In the future I will be able to do most of the same   SA A U D SD
    things I did before I got sick.
43. Until I am better I may have trouble asking other   SA A U D SD
    people to do things for me (for example, buying
    groceries).
44. I understand what kinds of food I can eat.   SA A U D SD
45. Sometimes I worry about having another heart   SA A U D SD
    attack.
46. Making some changes in the things I do may help   SA A U D SD
    prevent me from having this kind of illness again.

Part B

Directions: All of the statements in this Part B (47 through 60) also refer
to how you are feeling now but there are six possible responses to each
of the statements. They are:

               SA = Strongly Agree
               A = Agree
               U = Uncertain
               D = Disagree
               SD = Strongly Disagree
               NA = Does Not Apply to me

For each statement, circle the letter(s) which best describes your feeling.

47. My partner (important person) has helped me to   SA A U D SD NA
    feel better about myself since I have been here.
48. My partner (important person), worries too   SA A U D SD NA
    much about me.
49. My partner (important person) understands how I SA A U D SD NA
    am feeling right now.
50. My partner (important person) will help me to   SA A U D SD NA
    make the changes in my everyday living that
    my doctor or nurse has suggested.

                                          Please go to the next page

Key: SA = Strongly Agree
      A = Agree
      U = Uncertain
      D = Disagree
      SD = Strongly Disagree
      NA = Does Not Apply to me

51. After my doctor says it is all right for me to resume sexual activities, my partner will be worried about that. SA A U D SD NA

52. My partner (important person) does not worry enough about me. SA A U D SD NA

53. When my doctor says it is all right, I believe I will be able to go back to work. SA A U D SD NA

54. I sometimes worry that I will not have enough money to take care of my expenses until I go back to work. SA A U D SD NA

55. My illness means that I might have to change my job. SA A U D SD NA

56. My illness means that I might lose my job. SA A U D SD NA

57. I understand why I am taking medicines. SA A U D SD NA

58. I understand what the unwanted side effects are of the medicines I am taking. SA A U D SD NA

59. I believe that if I am feeling all right that I can stop taking my medicines without asking my doctor or nurse. SA A U D SD NA

60. I understand that if unwanted side effects of my medicines happen, that I should report this to my doctor or nurse right away. SA A U D SD NA

THIS IS THE END OF THE SURVEY. IF YOU HAVE ANY COMMENTS TO MAKE ABOUT THE SURVEY. PLEASE WRITE THEM BELOW' OR ON THE BACK OF THIS PAGE.

THANK YOU FOR YOUR PARTICIPATION.

8

Schwartz Cancer Fatigue Scale

Anna L. Schwartz

This chapter discusses the Schwartz Cancer Fatigue Scale, a measure of cancer-related fatigue.

PURPOSE

Reliable and valid measures are critical to furthering our understanding of cancer-related fatigue (fatigue). Although the etiology of fatigue is unknown, researchers and clinicians are concerned with the evaluation and management of the symptom. Interest in fatigue has grown as the incidence (40%–100% of patients) and intensity of the symptom has been recognized (Irvine, Vincent, Bubela, & Thompson, 1991; Stetz, Haberman, Holcombe, Jones, & Moore, 1995). Methodological problems in the evaluation of cancer-related fatigue have hampered the ability of both researchers and clinicians to assess fatigue in cancer patients and develop interventions to treat and manage the symptom. Numerous measures of fatigue are available, but are embedded in scales intended to measure other constructs, are excessively lengthy, or lack adequate psychometric testing (Cella, 1997; McCorkle & Young, 1978; McNair, Lorr, & Droppleman, 1992; Piper, 1997; Piper, Lindsey, & Dodd, 1987). The Schwartz Cancer Fatigue Scale (SCFS) was developed specifically to measure cancer-related fatigue. It is a reliable, valid, and parsimonious, 6–item instrument that measures cancer-related fatigue on a physical and perceptual dimension.

CONCEPTUAL BASIS

Cancer-related fatigue is a symptom that negatively impacts normal activities, cognitive abilities, and quality of life (Massias, Yeager, Dibble, & Dodd, 1997; Nail & Jones, 1995; Nail & Winningham, 1995). Fatigue is a highly variable state that is characterized as unpredictable, varying widely throughout the day, and affected by type of treatment (Greene, Nail, Fieler, Dudgeon, & Jones, 1994). Cancer-related fatigue is a symptom that does not resolve when treatment stops and has been observed to linger years after treatment has ended (Fobair, Hope, & Bloom, 1986).

Substantive and theoretical research on cancer-related fatigue formed the basis for the development of the Schwartz Cancer Fatigue Scale (SCFS). Fatigue was conceptualized as a self-perceived state consisting of two dimensions: physical and perceptual. The physical dimension of fatigue includes components that may contribute to declines in physical function. The perceptual dimension is characterized by decreases in attention and changes in mood state that may affect action preparedness. The operational definition of fatigue that guided the development of the SCFS is one that defines it as a dynamic, multidimensional, self-perceived state.

A conceptual framework of fatigue initially evolved from a synthesis of Piper's Integrated Fatigue Model (Piper et al., 1987) and Cimprich's Attentional Fatigue Theory (Cimprich, 1992a, 1992b). As the scale was refined, the model of fatigue was more clearly specified. The model of fatigue proposes that cognitive fatigue may develop as a result of physical fatigue. The conceptual framework indicates that there is a direct relationship from the physical dimension to the perceptual dimension of fatigue. Being "overcome" by fatigue and experiencing "difficulty thinking" may be direct sequelae of physical fatigue or the result of an accumulation of fatigue, as proposed by Aistars' Organizing Framework (Aistars, 1987).

PROCEDURES FOR DEVELOPMENT

The SCFS was developed with attention to the theoretical constructs of fatigue and the perspective of the cancer patient's experience, specifically the physical and perceptual dimensions of fatigue. Seventy-two items were generated from an extensive review of the literature, self-report instruments, and words used by patients. Formal content validity was determined by patients and health care professionals following the guidelines proposed by Lynn (1986). Forty-one items met the criteria for retention.

A heterogeneous sample ($n = 166$) of cancer patients actively receiving treatment and cancer survivors who had completed treatment were used in the next phase of development (Schwartz, 1998a). Subjects ranged in age from 19 to 81 ($M = 48$, $SD = 11.8$) and were primarily male (66%), with a diversity of cancer diagnoses, stages of disease, and types of treatment. Subjects were asked to complete the 41–item SCFS and place a mark through a 100 mm single-item visual analogue scale of fatigue (VAS-F) to indicate how much fatigue they had experienced in the past two to three days. Items were eliminated that (1) had poor variance, (2) had high item-to-item correlations, (3) failed to discriminate between subjects on treatment and those who had completed treatment, and (4) failed to differentiate between groups on level of fatigue reported on the VAS-F. Factor analysis resulted in a four-factor solution accounting for 70% of the variance in fatigue. Internal consistency reliability was estimated by Cronbach's coefficient alpha to be .96 for the total scale. Cronbach's coefficient alpha for the subscales ranged from .82 to .93.

A second study tested the construct validity of the SCFS on a different sample of 303 heterogeneous cancer patients from across the United States (Schwartz & Meek, 2000). Subjects were primarily male (61%) and ranged in age from 19 to 81 ($M = 50$). Latent variable modeling was used to assess the hypothesized relationships between the measured variables and the latent construct proposed through goodness of fit indices. The four subscales proposed by the exploratory factor analysis were not supported and multiple variations of the model were tested with latent variable modeling using the generalized least-squares method. The strongest model proposed two factors with three items loading on a physical factor (factor 1) and three items on a perceptual factor (factor 2). All measures of fit were consistently strong ($> .92$) and all standardized solution factors loaded strongly ($> .73$). The total scale has excellent internal consistency reliability ($\alpha > .90$), as did the physical and perceptual subscales ($\alpha > .88$ and .81 respectively). Discriminate validity was determined using t-tests to differentiate between subjects who were currently receiving treatment and those who had completed treatment and by level of fatigue. Significant differences were observed by treatment group ($p < .000$ for all items) and by level of fatigue ($p < .001$ for all items, total fatigue score, and time since last treatment).

Two multisite repeated measures instrumentation trials were conducted. The first (Study 3) tested the psychometric properties of six different fatigue scales in 212 cancer patients receiving either chemotherapy or radiotherapy (Meek et al., 2000; Nail, 1998). Subjects completed the six scales when fatigue was expected to be highest (completion of radiation therapy or two days after chemotherapy) and again when fatigue was expected to be lower, either four weeks after the completion of radiation therapy or immediately prior to the next administration of chemotherapy. The mean age was 56.6 years. Subjects were predominately married (78%), female (57%), and breast cancer was the most frequent diagnosis (34%). Results demonstrated that the 6–item SCFS correlated strongly ($p < .01$) with other validated measures (Table 8.1). Coefficient alpha for the total scale was .89 and greater than .80 for the two subscales. Stability was examined over a two-day period in a subset of 37 subjects. Given the highly variable state of fatigue, the stability coefficients were reasonable (total scale $r = .69$, physical subscale $r = .75$, perceptual subscale $r = .63$). The SCFS was highly sensitive ($p < .001$) to change over the two-day time frame.

The magnitude of change in cancer-related fatigue as measured by the SCFS was examined over one cycle of chemotherapy or during the month

TABLE 8.1 Reliability and Validity Evidence for the SCFS

Study citation	Sample and characteristics	Reliability evidence	Validity evidence
1. Schwartz, A. L. (1998a). Reliability and validity of the Schwartz Cancer Fatigue Scale. *Oncology Nursing Forum, 25,* 711–719.	*Sample size:* 166. *Sample characteristics:* National survey. Sample from across U.S.A. Sample heterogeneous with respect to age, type and stage of cancer, and type of treatment. Sample included both patients receiving treatment and cancer survivors.	*Cronbach's alpha for total scale and subscales* Total Scale .97 Physical Subscale .93 Emotional Subscale .90 Cognitive Subscale .85 Temporal Subscale .82	A priori and formal content validity conducted. Results of factor analysis for the SCFS total scale. *Factor / Subscale / Eigenvalue / %Variance / Cumulative %* 1 Physical 15.31 54.7 54.7 2 Emotional 1.61 5.7 60.4 3 Cognitive 1.43 5.1 65.5 4 Temporal 1.26 4.5 70.0
2. Schwartz, A., & Meek, P. (2000). Additional content validity of the Schwartz Cancer Fatigue Scale. *Journal of Nursing Measurement, 7,* 35–45. Schwartz, A. L., Meek, P. M., Nail, L. M., Berendts, C., Grainger, M., Throckmorton, T., Mateo, M., Fargo, J., & Lundquist,	*Sample size:* 303. *Sample characteristics:* Heterogeneous sample obtained by survey. Sample differed with respect to type and stage of cancer, type of treatment and duration of treatment.	*Cronbach's alpha for total scale and subscales* Total Scale .90 Physical .88 Perceptual .81	*Results of latent variable modeling for the six item SCFS.* Chi-square 147.267 with 15df; $p > .05$ Bentler-Bonnett Normed .92 Comparative Fit Index (CFI) .95 Liseral GFI .99 Liseral AGFI .95 *Item loadings on each factor.* **Item** / **Factor 1** / **Factor 2** Worn-out .93 Tired .80

TABLE 8.1 (*continued*)

Study citation	Sample and characteristics	Reliability evidence	Validity evidence
M. (2000). Fatigue patterns of chemotherapy (CT) naïve (N), experienced (E) & Recurrent(R) patients. *Program/proceedings American Society of Clinical Oncology, 19,* 645a.			Listless .76 Difficulty thinking .75 Overcome .84 Helpless .73 *Discriminant validity* T-tests between those receiving and completed treatment ($p < .000$ for all items). <table><tr><td></td><td colspan="2">Receiving treatment</td><td colspan="2">Completed treatment</td></tr><tr><td></td><td>Mean</td><td>SD</td><td>Mean</td><td>SD</td></tr><tr><td>Total scale</td><td>14.5</td><td>5.4</td><td>8.8</td><td>3.5</td></tr><tr><td>Physical</td><td>8.4</td><td>3.0</td><td>4.9</td><td>2.1</td></tr><tr><td>Perceptual</td><td>6.1</td><td>2.8</td><td>3.9</td><td>1.6</td></tr></table>
3. Meek, P. M., Nail, L. M., Barsevick, A., Schwartz, A. L., Stephens, S., Whitmer, K., Beck, S. L., Jones, L., & Walker, B. L. (2000). Psychometric testing of fatigue instruments for use with cancer treatment-patients. *Nursing Research, 49,* 181–190.	*Sample size:* 212 *Sample characteristics:* Multisite study of diverse sample of adults receiving chemotherapy for a variety of types and stages of cancer.	*Cronbach's alpha for total scale and subscales* Total Scale .89 Physical .88 Perceptual .80 *Stability coefficient* Total Scale $r = .69$ Physical $r = .75$ Perceptual $r = .63$	*SCFS Correlations with other measures ($p < .01$ all scales):* Profile of Mood States Total scale $r = .71$ Profile of Mood State Fatigue subscale $r = .83$ Lee's Fatigue Scale $r = .63$ Multidimensional Fatigue Inventory $r = -.68$ Multidimensional Assessment of Fatigue $r = .79$ General Fatigue Scale $r = .77$ *Effect size by GLM model = 0.98* *Sensitivity to change over 2 day period $t = 4.16$, $r < .001$*

TABLE 8.1 (continued)

Study citation	Sample and characteristics	Reliability evidence	Validity evidence
4. Schwartz, A. L., Meek, P. M., Nail, L. M., fargo, J., Lundquist, M., Donofrio, M., Grainger, M., Throckmorton, T., Mateo, M. (2002). Measurement of fatigue: Determining minimally important clinical differences. *Journal of Clinical Epidemiology, 55*, 239–244.	*Sample size:* 123 *Sample characteristics:* Multisite study of inpatient or outpatient adults with cancer receiving chemotherapy or bone marrow transplant.	*Cronbach's alpha for total scale and subscales* Total Scale .90 Physical .89 Perceptual .82	*Clinically important differences* Small Mean change = 3.9 ± 4.1 Moderate Mean change = 6.4 ± 4.9 Large Mean change = 8.0 ± 5.3 *Effect size* = .71 *Sensitivity to change over 2 day period t* = 6.77, *r* < .001

following the completion of radiation therapy in a subset of subjects from Study 3. Subjects (N = 73) were middle aged (M = 52.4 ± 14.2), female (67%), and receiving either chemotherapy (N = 51) or radiation therapy (N = 22). The mean change from the high point (end of radiation therapy or 2 days post-chemotherapy) to the low point (28 days post-radiation therapy and before the next dose of chemotherapy) was 2.5 (± 5.18). Scores for the high point of treatment for the total group ranged from 6 to 29 (M = 15.03 ± 5.64). Scores for the low point ranged from 7 to 26 (M = 12.5 ± 4.91). The observed effect size for the mean change was .98 computed by the GLM effect size model (Schwartz, 1998b).

The purpose of the second multisite study (Study 4) was to determine the minimally important clinical difference in fatigue, or the smallest amount of change in fatigue that is clinically important. Using the methods of Jaeschke and colleagues (1989), a multisite repeated measures design trial of 123 cancer patients receiving chemotherapy was conducted. Subjects were asked to complete the 6–item SCFS and rate the amount of change in their fatigue over a two–day period as *no change, a little change, moderate change,* or *large change.* Subjects represented diverse types and stages of cancer. The majority of subjects (60%) were female, middle aged (M = 50 years ± 17), and all were receiving chemotherapy. The minimally important clinical difference (small amount of change in fatigue) for the SCFS was a mean change of 3.9 points (± 4.1). Moderate and large changes in fatigue were found to be a mean change of 6.4 (± 4.9) and 8.0 (± 5.3), respectively. In this sample, the effect size for the SCFS was observed to be .70. For a researcher, these results may be useful when calculating sample size requirements and interpreting results in clinically meaningful terms. For clinicians, the ability to estimate clinically important differences in fatigue is essential in interpreting studies that show statistically significant findings.

DESCRIPTION

The brief, six–item scale assesses cancer-related fatigue on a physical and perceptual dimension. Each subscale has three items. The total scale provides an overall assessment of fatigue, while the subscales allow clinicians and researchers to differentiate between physical and perceptual fatigue and direct interventions that are specific to the type of fatigue experienced. The scale is found at the end of this chapter in the Appendix.

ADMINISTRATION AND SCORING

The SCFS can be self-administered or read to the respondent. Respondents circle a number from 1 = *not at all* to 5 = *extremely.* Scores for the total scale are derived by summing all six items. Scores for the total scale range from 6 to 30 with higher scores denoting greater fatigue. The subscale scores are derived by summing the individual items on each subscale. Items on the physical subscale are *worn-out, tired* and *listless.* Items on the perceptual subscale are *difficulty thinking, helpless,* and *overcome.* Scores for each of the subscales range from 3 to 15, with higher scores indicating greater levels of physical or perceptual fatigue.

RELIABILITY AND VALIDITY

The evidence for reliability and validity for the SCFS from each of the four psychometric studies are displayed in Table 8.1.

CONCLUSIONS AND RECOMMENDATIONS

The SCFS is a parsimonious measure of cancer-related fatigue that may prove useful in both clinical and research settings. The six–item, two-dimensional model of the SCFS is supported by results of confirmatory factor analysis and strong internal consistency reliability. The development of the SCFS is grounded in knowledge of substantive and theoretical research in cancer-related fatigue to specify the best fitting model. The SCFS is psychometrically strong with excellent content validity, reliability, and evidence of construct and discriminant validity. Unlike most measures of cancer-related fatigue, which are incorporated in instruments intended to measure other aspects of functioning, the SCFS is the only brief measure developed specifically to measure the fatigue of cancer and its treatment. The brevity and multidimensionality of this instrument makes it attractive for use with a population of patients known to be affected by fatigue. The preliminary work on establishing the clinically important difference in fatigue may be important to help researchers determine effect size and calculate sample size, and help clinicians assess fatigue and monitor responses to treatment.

The SCFS has been widely adopted nationally and internationally. It has been translated into different languages (e.g. Chinese, Korean) and is currently undergoing psychometric testing in these languages. The SCFS is also being tested and used with different patient populations (e.g., those with rheumatoid arthritis, chronic obstructive pulmonary disease, diabetes, hepatitis C). The translated versions and the reliability and validity from these different studies are not available at this time.

The primary limitation of the SCFS is that it has not been tested in time frames other than "in the past two to three days." Further research is needed to examine the psychometrics of the scale using different time frames that might be useful to researchers and clinicians (e.g., in the past month). Additional testing is also needed to further assess discriminate and construct validity of the two dimensional SCFS. Other psychometric studies should evaluate the ability of the SCFS to measure fatigue in pediatric patients and in other disease states where fatigue is problematic.

REFERENCES

Aistars, J. (1987). Fatigue in the cancer patients: A conceptual approach to a clinical problem. *Oncology Nursing Forum, 12,* 122–127.

Cella, D. (1997). The Functional Assessment of Cancer Therapy-Anemia (FACT-An) Scale: A new tool for the assessment of outcome in cancer anemia and fatigue. *Seminars in Hematology, 34,* (Suppl. 2), 13–19.

Cimprich, B. (1992a). A theoretical perspective on attention and patient education. *Advances in Nursing Science, 14,* 39–51.

Cimprich, B. (1992b). Attentional fatigue following breast cancer surgery. *Research in Nursing & Health, 15,* 199–207.

Fobair, P., Hope, R. T., & Bloom, L. (1986). Psychosocial problems among survivors of Hodgkin's disease. *Journal of Clinical Oncology, 4,* 805–814.

Greene, D., Nail, L. M., Fieler, V., Dudgeon, B., & Jones, L. S. (1994). A comparison of patient reported side effects among three chemotherapy regimens for breast cancer. *Cancer Practice, 2,* 57–62.

Irvine, D.M., Vincent, L., Bubela, N., & Thompson, L. (1991). A critical appraisal of the research literature investigating fatigue in cancer patients. *Cancer Nursing ,14,* 188–199.

Jaeschke, R., Singer, J., & Guyatt, G. H. (1989). Measurement of health status: Ascertaining the minimal clinically important difference. *Controlled Clinical Trials, 1,* 407–415.

Lynn, M. R. (1986). Determination and quantification of content validity. *Nursing Research, 35,* 382–385.

Massias, D. K. H., Yeager, K. A., Dibble, S. L., & Dodd, M. J. (1997). Patients' perspectives of fatigue while undergoing chemotherapy. *Oncology Nursing Forum, 24,* 43–48.

McCorkle, R., & Young, K. (1978). Development of a symptom distress scale. *Cancer Nursing, 5,* 373–378.

McNair,D. M., Lorr, M., & Droppleman, L. F. (1992). *Profile of Mood States manual.* San Diego: CA Educational and Industrial Testing Service.

Meek, P. M., Nail, L. M., Barsevick, A., Schwartz, A. L., Stephens, S., Whitmer, K., Beck, S. L., Jones, L., Walker, B. L. (2000). Psychometric testing of fatigue instruments for use with cancer patients. *Nursing Research, 49,* 181–190.

Nail, L. M. (1998). [Fatigue initiative in research and education phase I instrumentation grant]. Unpublished raw data. University of Utah

Nail, L. M., & Jones, L. S. (1995). Fatigue as a side effect of cancer treatment: Impact on quality of life. *Quality of Life—A Nursing Challenge, 4,* 8–13.

Nail, L. M., & Winningham, M. L. (1995). Fatigue and weakness in cancer patients: The symptom experience. *Seminars in Oncology Nursing, 11,* 272–278.

Piper, B. F. (1997). Measuring fatigue. In M. Frank-Stromborg & S. J. Olsen (Eds.), *Instruments for clinical health-care research* (pp. 482–496). Boston: Jones and Bartlett.

Piper, B., Lindsey, A., & Dodd, M. (1987). Fatigue mechanisms in cancer patients: Developing nursing theory. *Oncology Nursing Forum, 14,* 17–23.

Schwartz, A. L. (1998a). Reliability and validity of the Schwartz Cancer Fatigue Scale. *Oncology Nursing Forum, 25,* 711–719.

Schwartz, A. L. (1998b, January). *Overall change in cancer treatment-related fatigue as measured by the Schwartz Cancer Fatigue Scale (SCFS).* Proceedings from the Nursing Research Conference: Research for Clinical Practice, School of Nursing, University of Arizona, Tucson.

Schwartz, A., & Meek, P. (2000). Additional content validity of the Schwartz Cancer Fatigue Scale. *Journal of Nursing Measurement, 7,* 35–45.

Schwartz, A. L., Meek, P. M., Nail, L. M., Berendts, C., Grainger, M., Throckmorton, T., Mateo, M., Fargo, J., Lundquist, M. (2000). Fatigue patterns of chemotherapy (CT) naïve (N), experienced (E) & Recurrent (R) patients. *Program/Proceedings American Society of Clinical Oncology, 19,* 645a.

Schwartz, A. L., Meek, P. M., Nail, L. M., Fargo, J., Lundquist, M., Donofrio, M., Grainger, M., Throckmorton, T., Mateo, M. (2002). Measurement of fatigue: Determining minimally important clinical differences. *J. Clinical Epidemiology, 55,* 239–244.

Stetz, K., Haberman, M., Holcombe, J., Jones, L., & Moore, K. (1995). 1994 Oncology Nursing Society Research Priorities Survey, *Oncology Nursing Forum, 22,* 785–789.

APPENDIX: SCHWARTZ CANCER FATIGUE SCALE (SCFS-6)

The words and phrases below describe different feelings people associate with fatigue. Please read each item and circle the number that indicates how much fatigue has made you feel in the past 2 to 3 days.

1 = not at all
2 = a little
3 = moderately
4 = quite a bit
5 = extremely

Tired	1	2	3	4	5
Difficulty thinking	1	2	3	4	5
Overcome	1	2	3	4	5
Listless	1	2	3	4	5
Worn out	1	2	3	4	5
Helpless	1	2	3	4	5

9

ADL Self-Care Scale for Persons with Multiple Sclerosis

Elsie E. Gulick

This chapter describes the 55- and 15-item ADL Self-Care Scales (ADL-MS), which were designed to assess the ability of persons with multiple sclerosis (MS) to undertake activities of daily living (ADL) for self-care.

PURPOSE

The ADL Self-Care Scales (ADL-MS) consist of long and short forms, which assess the ability of persons with MS to undertake self-care operations on a daily basis. The 55-item ADL-MS was factored into 6 subscales: Upper Body (dressing, bathing, transfer, eating), Lower Body (walking, travel), Intimacy, Recreation and Socializing, Sensory and Communication, and Bowel Elimination. Refactoring of the original 55-item ADL-MS for reasons of parsimony resulted in 15 items among 4 factored subscales: Motor (eating, dressing, bathing, walking, travel), Intimacy, Sensory and Communication, and Recreation and Socializing. These scales can be used with persons diagnosed with multiple sclerosis (MS) to monitor their health, and can be useful to nurses and other health providers for the evaluation of treatment outcomes and research on MS.

CONCEPTUAL BASIS OF THE ADL SELF-CARE SCALE FOR PERSONS WITH MULTIPLE SCLEROSIS

Self-care, the practice of activities that individuals initiate and perform on their own behalf in maintaining life, health, and well-being, contributes to human structural integrity, human functioning, and human development (Orem, 1980, 1991). Orem has identified three categories of self-care requisites, namely, universal, developmental, and health-deviation. Universal requisites include maintaining sufficient intakes of air,

125

water, and food; provision for eliminative processes; maintenance of a balance between activity and rest and between solitude and social interaction; prevention of hazards to life, functioning, and well-being; and promotion of normalcy. Developmental self-care requisites include life transitions such as marriage, birth of a baby, and poor health or disability. Health deviation requisites exist for persons who are ill or injured, have specific defects and disabilities, or who are undergoing diagnosis and/or treatment. Self-care deficits occur when individuals are unable to manage their self-care requisites either partially or completely, resulting in dependency and the need for assistance or total care from health professionals and/or family.

Orem (1991) posits a number of propositions pertaining to self-care in health and disease. First, self-care contributes to and is necessary for a person's integrity as a psychophysiologic organism with a rational life. Second, each person must perform or have performed for him/her each day a minimum of activities to continue existence as an organism with a rational life as well as perform additional activities when mental or physical malfunctioning is present. Third, self-care directed to the maintenance and promotion of health requires a scientifically derived fund of knowledge about self-care practices. Fourth, the presence of disease, injury, and mental or physical malfunctioning may limit what one can do for oneself due to structural and/or functional changes that may necessitate use of specialized self-care measures and services.

According to Orem (1991), performance of self-care activities requires three operations: estimative, transitional, and productive. Estimative operations require an investigation of internal and external conditions significant to self-care. Transitional operations involve reflection on which course of self-care is to be taken. Productive operations involve the preparation of self, materials, or environmental settings for undertaking self-care, and implementing and monitoring the chosen course. The ADL-MS scale was developed to assess the ability of persons with MS to undertake these self-care operations. Information obtained from these scales can be used by nurses and other health professionals in caring for their MS patients to determine the effectiveness of prescribed treatment outcomes in maintaining or increasing functional levels and in monitoring the patient's chronic illness trajectory.

PROCEDURES FOR DEVELOPMENT

The unavailability of a standardized (Keith, 1984), sensitive (Jeffreys, Millard, Human, & Warren, 1969; Kaufert, 1983) and self-administered ADL scale for use by persons with MS and/or their families led to the development of the 55-item ADL-MS (Gulick, 1988a). Initially, an attempt was undertaken to modify the Social Dependency Scale (McCorkle & Benoliel, 1981) by altering the existing Guttman-type statements in a manner that would reflect relevant ADL functions of persons with MS. However, the time required for staff administration and scoring of the ADL scale using the Guttman-type format led to recasting the items into a matrix-type scale that could be self-administered and easily scored by persons with MS or health professionals.

A number of guidelines were established in selecting items that would ensure content validity of the ADL-MS (Gulick, 1988a). These included the inclusion of essential activities encountered by all persons in everyday life that were especially important to persons with MS; determination of what functions the person with MS *presently performs,* not what the person *can perform,* together with the frequency with which those functions are performed; determination of those functions for which the person requires help from others and the frequency with which that help is received; scale sensitivity toward changing functional abilities; and self-administration or scale administration by a family member.

Items for the ADL-MS were obtained primarily from the experiences of client service personnel in their service to persons with MS through local chapters of the National Multiple Sclerosis Society located in New Jersey, through a review of the MS literature, and direct input by five persons who were in various phases of the MS illness trajectory. Changes in ADL items were made until three client service workers, this author, and five MS clients agreed that the items were representative of ADL encountered by persons with MS, thus providing content validity of the ADL-MS.

The 55-item ADL-MS, containing 11 subscales for *self-care* (Dressing, Bathing, Transfer, Eating, Walking, Travel, Intimacy, Recreation and Socializing, Sensory and Communication, Bowel Elimination, Urine Elimination), are repeated to determine the person's receipt of *help from others* except for the Intimacy subscale (Gulick, 1988a). The scale was pilot tested among 28 persons with MS who averaged 51.6 years of age, 13.4 years of education, and 13.7 years since being diagnosed with MS. Seventy-five percent of the sample were women. Cronbach alpha reliability coefficients for the Self-Care subscales ranged between .60 and .98, with the exception of the subscales Walking, Sensory and Communication, and Intimacy. Stability coefficients ranged between .66 and .91. Cronbach alpha reliability coefficients for the *Help from Others* subscales ranged between .77 and .97 and the stability correlation coefficient range was .33 to .91. The subscales Walking, Sensory and Communication, and Intimacy were subsequently reviewed, revised, and accepted as part of the 55-item ADL-MS.

DESCRIPTION

The 55-item ADL-MS consists of 11 subscales (Eating, Dressing, Bathing, Transfer, Walking, Travel, Intimacy, Recreation and Socializing, Sensory

and Communication, Toileting-Urination, Toileting-Bowel) each containing five items that measure self-care ability. These subscales, except for
Intimacy, are repeated for determining help received from others in performing the respective activities. Factor analysis of the 55-item ADL-MS
resulted in six factors: *Upper Body* (Eating, Dressing, Bathing, and Transfer subscales), *Lower Body* (Walking and Travel subscales). *Intimacy, Recreation and Socializing, Sensory and Communication* and *Bowel Elimination*. The
Urination subscale failed to emerge as a factor and was again revised as a
separate subscale and tested on a sample of 94 additional persons with
MS, yielding a Cronbach alpha of .71. Refactoring of the 55-item ADL-MS
scale for purposes of parsimony resulted in four factors, which comprise
the 15-item ADL-MS: Motor, Intimacy, Sensory and Communication, and
Recreation and Socializing. All items in the ADL-MS use a six-point Likert-type rating format from 0 (*Never*) to 5 (*Always*).

ADMINISTRATION AND SCORING

The 55-item and a 15-item ADL-MS scales can be self-administered by the
person with MS independently or, if needed, can be assisted by a family
member, or health personnel can obtain the information through client
interview. Respondents are asked to rate each *Self-Care* item according to
how frequently he/she performs the behavior on a typical day. For the
55-item Self-Care Scale only, ratings are reverse scored for all items in the
Urination and Bowel Elimination subscales and the fifth item, "Transfer
only with assistance of mechanical devices such as a patient lift" in the
Transfer subscale to reflect positive or less invasive self-care behavior. The
five items contained within each of the 11 subscales can be summed to
yield total subscale scores between 0 and 25, where higher scores suggest
a higher level of ADL functioning. In rating the items contained within
each of the 10 *Help from Others* subscales respondents are asked to make
ratings according to how much help from others they receive for each
behavior. The latter scores are summed to yield total subscale scores
between 0 and 25, where higher scores indicate increased dependency
needs. Subjects can graph their own MS Self-Care ADL Profile by placing
Self-Care and *Help from Others* subscale scores on a grid. The short and
long forms of the ADL Self-Care Scale will be found in the Appendix at
the end of this chapter, along with the self-scoring grid. Difference scores
can be obtained by subtracting *Help from Others* subscale scores from *Self-
Care* subscale scores. Positive difference scores suggest greater independence in performing ADL and negative scores suggest greater dependency
on other persons to perform those activities. All items contained within
the 15-item ADL scale can be summed to yield a total score between 0
and 75 where higher scores suggest a higher level of functioning. Summing over the 12 items in the *Help from Others* scale yields a score range

between 0 and 60. To facilitate comparisons among factored subscales within the 55-item and 15-item ADL-MS scales, one should sum the item ratings for the respective subscale and divide by the number of items to yield a score between 0 and 5. Administration time is approximately 30 minutes for the 55-item scale and about five minutes for the 15-item scale.

RELIABILITY AND VALIDITY EVIDENCE

Evidence for stability and internal consistency and for a priori content validity, together with construct and criterion-related validity are shown in Tables 9.1 and 9.2 for the total and subscales of the 55- and 15-item ADL-MS scales, respectively. Most study samples consisted of persons with MS but a sample of spinal cord injured and stroke patients are also reported.

CONCLUSIONS AND RECOMMENDATIONS

Consistent with Orem's (1980, 1991) self-care conceptual framework, the availability of self-assessment scales that measure what ADL behaviors the person with chronic illness perform and those that require help from others is essential in today's health care environment. Reliable and valid self-assessment scales encourage and even may force families to shoulder increasing responsibility for the individual's health care needs. The 55- and 15-item ADL-MS scales provide individuals with MS and their families a mechanism that captures behavioral actions essential for estimating Orem's universal self-care requisites pertaining to intake of water and food; provision for eliminative processes, activity, and social interaction; and promotion of normalcy. The ADL-MS identifies health deviation requisites that are common to persons with MS and to persons with other neurological illnesses such as spinal cord injury and stroke. Data obtained from the ADL-MS scales provide the individual with information about his/her internal and external conditions that are significant to meeting self and/or dependent care requirements.

As shown in Tables 9.1 and 9.2, the 55- and 15-item ADL-MS scales have undergone considerable reliability and validity testing by this author and others. Satisfactory test–retest reliability indicates good stability and both theta and Cronbach alpha reliability coefficients indicate good internal consistency for the total and subscales. A priori internal consistency and construct and criterion-related validity testing over many studies suggest good validity of the total and subscales.

The ADL-MS scales can be used for determining the effectiveness of particular treatments and/or interventions, and in monitoring changes

TABLE 9.1 Reliability and Validity of the 55-item ADL Self-Care Scale

Study citation	Sample and characteristics	Reliability evidence	Validity evidence
Gulick, E. E. (1988a). The self-administered scale for persons with multiple sclerosis. In C. F. Waltz & O. L. Strickland (Eds.), *Measurement of nursing outcomes: Vol. 1: Measuring client outcomes* (pp. 128–159). New York: Springer.	*Sample size:* 629 adults with MS. *Characteristics:* Persons diagnosed with MS averaging 48.5 years of age, 12.6 years since diagnosis, 12.5 years of education. 75% were women and 45% had one or more pre- or school-age children.	*Self-Care Scale:* *Test-retest:* 2–3 week period Total scale r = .86 Factored subscales r's ranged between .73 and .93. *Internal Consistency:* Total scale α = .96 Upper Body subscale θ = .97 Lower Body subscale θ = .95 Intimacy subscale θ = .91 Recreation & Socializing θ = .86 Sensory & Communication θ = .75 Bowel Elimination subscale θ = .63 Urination subscale α = .71 *Help from Others Scale* *Test-retest:* 1–3 week period Total scale r = .92 Factored subscales r's ranged between .72 and .92 *Internal Consistency:* Total scale α = .97.	*Self-Care Scale:* *A priori content validity:* Items were generated from MS client service workers, MS clients, and review of literature. *Construct validity:* Exploratory factor analysis with orthogonal rotation extracted 6 factors. Factor names and factor range of factor loadings were: Upper Body (.38 to .90), Lower Body (.39 to .81), Intimacy (.52 to .93), Recreation & Socializing (.61 to .76), Sensory & Communication (.35 to .64), Bowel elimination (.35 to .74). *Criterion-related concurrent validity:* Factored ADL subscale scores were correlated with factored scores obtained from the MS-Related Symptom Scale (Gulick, 1988a) as follows: Upper Body, Lower Body, Recreation & Socializing, Sensory & communication and Bowel Elimination correlated with Motor symptoms (r's = –.37, –.46, –.34, –.35, –.23); Recreation & Socializing and Sensory & Communication also correlated with Brainstem (r's = –.22, –.23) and Mental/Emotion (r's = –.38, –.23) symptoms.

TABLE 9.1 (*continued*)

Study citation	Sample and characteristics	Reliability evidence	Validity evidence
Gulick, E. E. (1988b). Concurrent validity for the ADL Self-Care Scale. *Proceedings of the national symposium of nursing research: Promoting quality of patient care through research* (pp. 91–95). San Francisco, CA.	*Sample size:* 70 adults from a MS outpatient clinic and 60 from a local National MS chapter. *Characteristics:* Persons diagnosed with MS averaging for the respective samples 47.4 and 47.8 years of age, and 11.7 and 11.7 years since diagnosis.		*SelfCare Scale* *Criterion-related concurrent validity:* Factored ADL subscale scores were correlated with the Kurtzke Disability Status Scale (DSS) (International Federation of MS Societies, 1984) and the Incapacity Status Scale (ISS) (International Federation of MS Societies, 1985) as follows. ADL Subscale — DDS / ISS Upper Body −.61 / −.84 Lower Body −.79 / −.84 Intimacy −.27 / −.21 Rec. & Soc. −.47 / −.57 Sens. & Comm. −.36 / −.28 Urination −.28 / −.28 Bowel Elim. −.11 / −.17 Total ADL −.75 / −.89
Gulick, E. G. (1991b). Reliability and validity of the Work Assessment Scale for Persons with Multiple Sclerosis. *Nursing Research, 40*(2), 107–112.	*Sample size:* 551 adults with MS *Characteristics:* In years S's averaged 49.7 for age, 14.6 for duration of MS, and 13.4 for education. 74% were females, 24.5% employed, 35.2% homemakers, 15.4% unemployed, 5.3% disabled, 13.6% retired.	*Internal Consistency:* Theta reliability coefficients ranged between .71 and .97 for 4 subscales used in the study: Upper Body, Lower Body, Recreation & Socializing, Sensory & Communication.	*Criterion-related concurrent validity:* Pearson correlation coefficients depicting relationships between Work Impediment subscales (Mobility, Hand Functions, Environmental Barriers, Heavy Labor) of the Work Assessment Scale and ADL-MS factors ranged between −.24 and −.53. Correlations between the Personal Attributes subscale of the Work Enhancers scale ranged between .18 and .33 and for Environmental Adjustment subscale was −.15 to −.40.

TABLE 9.1 *(continued)*

Study citation	Sample and characteristics	Reliability evidence	Validity evidence
Gulick, E. E. (1991a). Self-assessed health and use of health services. *Western Journal of Nursing Research,* 13(2), 195–219.	*Sample size:* 49 experimental and 49 control MS s's matched on age, duration of MS, walking ability, and sex recruited from local National MS chapters. *Characteristics:* S's averaged 47 years of age, 11.7 years since MS diagnosis, and 71% were women.	*Internal consistency.** Upper Body subscale α = .98 Lower Body subscale α = .96 Rec. & Soc. Subscale α = .87 Sen. & Comm. Subscale α = .76 Bowel Elim. subscale α = .53 Urine Elim. subscale α = .68 Walking subscale α = .91	*Self-Care Scale* *Construct validity:* Experimental s's who conducted self-assessments of their ADL and symptoms over a 27-month period had significantly fewer hospitalizations than control s's who did not conduct self-assessments of their ADL and symptoms.
Robinson-Smith, G. (1993). Coping and life satisfaction after stroke. *Journal of Stroke and Cerebrovascular Diseases, 3,* 209–215.	*Sample size:* 73 marital pairs living at home, one of whom had a documented stroke in the last 6 to 12 months. *Characteristics:* Ages ranged between 55 and 80 years with a mean of 70.3. 92% were Caucasian and 70% of stroke clients were male.	*Internal consistency* (alpha) * Subscale Self Help Upper body .96 .96 Eating .84 .84 Dressing .95 .95 Bathing .94 .93 Transfer .84 .69 Lower body .92 .86 Walking .90 .80 Travel .97 .86	

TABLE 9.1 (continued)

Study citation	Sample and characteristics	Reliability evidence	Validity evidence
Wineman, N. M., Durand, E. J., & Steiner, R. P. (1994). A comparative analysis of coping behaviors in persons with multiple sclerosis or a spinal cord injury. *Research in Nursing and Health, 17*, 185–194.	*Sample:* 433 adults with MS and 257 adults with spinal cord injury. *Characteristics:* S's for the respective samples averaged 49 and 41 years of age, women comprised 75% and 22%, 7% and 21% had less than a high school education, 86.3% and 69.2% were Caucasian.	*Internal consistency:* Cronbach alpha was .94 for the total *Self Care* scale and was .96 for the total *Help from Others* scale for both samples.	
Flensner, G. (1999). The cooling-suit: a study of ten multiple sclerosis patients' experiences in daily life. *Journal of Advanced Nursing, 29*, 1444–1453.	*Sample size:* 10 (7 female, 3 male). *Characteristics:* Female and male s's averaged 46 and 49 years of age, and 13.5 and 11.3 years since their MS diagnosis.		*Construct validity:* S's wearing cooling suits covering the upper body and head for 30–40 minutes, 3–4 times a day for 4 weeks compared ADL functioning at baseline and 4 weeks later. Summated scores over the 11 subscales showed increased self-care ability from +6 to +51 with an average of +23.5, and decreased self-care ability from –2 to –24, with an average of –5. Most improvement was shown for Walking, Urine Elimination, and Rec. & Soc. activities.

*Unpublished data.

TABLE 9.2 Reliability and Validity of the 15-item ADL Self-Care Scale

Study citation	Sample and characteristics	Reliability evidence	Validity evidence
Gulick, E. E. (1987). Parsimony and model confirmation of the ADL Self-Care Scale for MS persons. *Nursing Research, 36*(5), 278–283.	*Sample size:* 629 adults with MS *Characteristics:* S's averaged 48.4 years of age, 12.5 years since diagnosis, and 13.2 years of education. 75% were female and 45% had one or more pre- or school-age children.	*Test–retest:* 2–4 week period between testing for 89 s's was .86 for total scale and ranged between .73 and .93 for the factored subscales. *Internal consistency:* Cronbach alpha for the total *Self-Care* scale was .96 and theta reliability coefficients for the subscales were Motor (0.91), Intimacy (.75), Sens. & Comm. (073), Recreation & Socializing (.88).	*A priori* content validity: Items were generated from MS client service workers, MS clients, and review of literature. *Construct validity:* Confirmatory factor analysis with 4 factors. Factor names and factor range of factor loadings were: Motor (.60 to .83), Intimacy (.74 to .90), Sens. & Comm. (.63 to .80), Rec. & Soc. (.83 to .88).
Gulick, E. E. (1992). Model for predicting work performance among persons with multiple sclerosis. *Nursing Research, 41*(5), 266–272.	*Sample size:* 201 adults with MS. *Characteristics:* In years average for age was 47.4, MS duration 11.0, education 13.8. 75% were female, 68% married, 35.5% employed, 29.1% homemakers, 15.7% retired, 3% disabled.	*Internal consistency:* Total ADL-MS Cronbach alpha was .91.	
Gulick, E. E., & Bugg, A. (1992). Holistic health	*Sample size:* 211 adults with MS. *Characteristics:* Cohort groups	*Internal consistency:* Cronbach alphas for the 5th of 5	*Construct validity:* Significant ADL decrements occurred

TABLE 9.2 (*continued*)

Study citation	Sample and characteristics	Reliability evidence	Validity evidence
patterning in multiple sclerosis. *Research in Nursing and Health, 15,* 175–185.	were formed based on length of MS since diagnosis accordingly: Group 1 (0–5 years), Group 2 (> 5 and ≤10 years), Group 3 (> 10 years). Average age for respective groups was 42.0, 44.2, and 52.6 and average education was 12.7, 13.5, and 13.6.	annual ADL *Self-Care* assessments were Motor (.92), Intimacy (.75), Sen. & Comm. (.70), Rec. & Soc. (.88).	within each group over the 5-year assessment period for Motor activities and within Groups 1 & 2 for Intimacy activities.
Gulick, E. E., Cook, S. D., & Troiano, R. (1993). Comparison of patient and staff assessment of MS patients' health status. *Acta Neurol. Scand. 88,* 87–93.	*Sample size:* 140 MS outpatients. *Characteristics:* S's averaged 41.7 years of age, 6.9 years since MS diagnosis, and 13.5 years of education. 77% were women, 71% White, 24% Black, and 5% Hispanic.		*Criterion-related concurrent validity:* Percent agreement based on ≤ 1 unit difference between patient's ADL and neurologists' Expanded Disability Status change scores over a 7–month period was 72%.
Gulick, E. E. (1994). Social support among persons with multiple sclerosis. *Research in Nursing and Health, 17,* 195–206.	*Sample size:* 200 adults with MS. *Characteristics:* S's averaged 47.4 years of age, 11 years since MS diagnosis, and 13.8 years of education. 75% were women.	*Internal consistency:* Cronbach alphas for the *Self-Care* subscales were: Motor (.92). Intimacy (.70), Sen. & Comm. (.77), Rec. & Soc. (.83), and was .91 for the total scale.	

TABLE 9.2 (*continued*)

Study citation	Sample and characteristics	Reliability evidence	Validity evidence
Gulick, E. E. (1995). Coping among spouses or significant others of persons with multiple sclerosis. *Nursing Research, 44,* 220–225.	*Sample size:* 156 spouse or significant others of persons with MS. *Characteristics:* S's averaged 48.3 years of age and 13.7 years of education. 61.3% were women, 78% were spouses and the remainder were mothers, sons, daughters, and friends.	*Internal consistency:* Cronbach alphas for the *Help from Others* subscales were: Motor (.90), Sen. & Comm. (.83), Rec. & Soc. (.94).	
Gulick, E. E. (1996). Health status, work impediments, and coping related to work roles of women with multiple sclerosis. *WORK: A Journal of Prevention, Assessment & Rehabilitation, 6,* 153–166.	*Sample size:* 408 women with MS. *Characteristics:* Cohort groups were formed based on age accordingly: Young (< 45 years), Middle-age (45–64 years).	*Internal consistency:* Cronbach alphas ranged between .72 and .92 for the *Self-Care* subscales.	*Construct validity:* Middle-age compared to Young women had significantly lower ADL functioning in Motor, Intimacy, Sens. & Comm. and Rec. & Soc. activities.
Gulick, E. E. (1997). Correlates of quality of life among persons with multiple sclerosis. *Nursing Research, 46,* 305–311.	*Sample size:* 153 adults with MS. *Characteristics:* S's averaged 57.4 years of age, 21.8 years since MS diagnosis, and 13.7 years of education. 68% were women.	*Internal consistency:* Cronbach alphas for the *Self-Care* subscales were: Motor (.93), Intimacy (.75), Sens. & Comm. (.84), Rec. & Soc. (.85).	

TABLE 9.2 (*continued*)

Study citation	Sample and characteristics	Reliability evidence	Validity evidence
Vickrey, B. G., Hays, R. D., Genovese, B. J., Myers, L. W., & Ellison, G. W. (1997). Comparison of a generic to disease-targeted health-related quality-of-life measures for multiple sclerosis. *J. Clin. Epidemiol.*, *50*, 557–569.	*Sample size:* 171 adults with MS. *Characteristics:* Average age was 45 and had MS 9.4 years. 72% were women, 60% married, 98% completed high school, 49% had a baccalaureate degree, 39% were currently working for pay.	*Test–retest:* 2-week interval Pearson *r*'s for 75 s's ranged between .64 and .88 for ADL *Self-Care* subscales and between .68 and .92 for *Help from Others* subscales. *Internal consistency:* Cronbach alphas for the Self-Care and *Help from Others* subscales were Motor (.95) Intimacy (.75), Sens. & Comm (.79, .83), Rec. & Soc. (.86, .94).	*Criterion Related Predictive Validity:* ADL *Self-Care Motor* subscale added significantly in explaining the variance in "symptom severity" and "ambulation status" over and above that explained by the SF-36. ADL *Help from Others* Sens. & Comm. subscale added significantly in explaining the variance in "Days unable to work or attend school in prior month" over and above that explained by the SF-36.
Gulick, E. E. (1998). Symptom and activities of daily living trajectory in multiple sclerosis: A 10-year study. *Nursing Research, 47* 137–146.	*Sample size:* 153 adults with MS. *Characteristics:* Cohort groups were formed based on length of MS since diagnosis accordingly: Group 1 (0–5 years), Group 2 (>5 and ≤ 10 years), Group 3 (> 10 years). Average age for respective groups was 51.6, 53.6, and 62.9 and average education was 12.7, 13.5, and 13.6.	*Internal consistency:* Cronbach alphas for the 10th of 10 annual ADL *Self-Care* assessments were Motor (.93), Intimacy (.75), Sen. & Comm. (.84), Rec. & Soc. (.85).	*Construct validity:* Significant ADL decrements occurred within each group over the 10-year assessment period for Motor, Sens. & Comm. and Rec. & Soc. activities and within Groups 1 & 2 for Intimacy activities.

TABLE 9.2 (*continued*)

Study citation	Sample and characteristics	Reliability evidence	Validity evidence
Gulick, E. E. (2001). Emotional distress and activities of daily living functioning in persons with multiple sclerosis. *Nursing Research, 50,* 147–154.	*Sample size:* 686 adults with MS. *Characteristics:* S's averaged 48.9 years of age, 13.1 years since MS diagnosis, and 13.5 years of education. 74.8% were women, and 35.4% were employed.	*Internal consistency:* Cronbach alpha for the total ADL *Self-Care* scale was .90.	*Construct validity:* The theorized inverse relationship between mental distress and ADL functioning was supported ($r = -.32$).

in health status over time. The 15-item scale can be used for rapid screening of the individual's overall independent and/or dependent functions pertaining to personal care, mobility, communication, and intimacy. However, the 55-item scale provides more detail regarding the latter areas as well as information pertaining to elimination processes that could be useful in planning interventions for specific individuals. The importance of making periodic health self-assessments using the ADL-MS scales, together with the receipt of ADL profiles depicting their functional level, was shown to significantly decrease hospitalizations among a group of persons with MS. MS patients who conducted annual health assessments had fewer hospitalizations compared to a matched control group who did not conduct self-assessments (Gulick, 1991a). It was reasoned that the subjects' self-assessment of their ADL functioning together with their ADL profiles, provided empirical knowledge from which they could make more accurate estimations of their health needs. In addition, they could more effectively evaluate the regulatory actions they had undertaken to determine whether particular health goals were achieved or if a new series of estimative operations should begin.

Although the ADL-MS scales were developed for use with persons with MS, the 55-item scale has been successfully used with two other neurologically impaired patient groups namely, Spinal Cord Injured and Stroke (Robinson-Smith, 1993; Wineman, Durand, & Steiner, 1994). Continued use of the ADL-MS is suggested for these groups. Further, Vickrey and colleagues (1997) strongly recommend using the MS-ADL Motor subscale in MS research when the SF-36 is chosen as a generic measure of health-related quality of life. Items in the Motor subscale "tend to tap physical health in a range that falls 'below' and complementary to functioning assessed by the SF-36 physical function scale" (p. 566). Thus, the ADL-MS scales warrant continued use in research and in guiding patients' self-care and care given to MS patients by nurses and other health care providers.

REFERENCES

Flensner, G. (1999). The cooling-suit: A study of ten multiple sclerosis patients' experiences in daily life. *Journal of Advanced Nursing 29*, 1444–1453.

Gulick, E. E., (1987). Parsimony and model confirmation of the ADL Self-Care scale for MS Persons. *Nursing Research, 36*, 278–283.

Gulick, E. E. (1988a). The self-administered ADL Scale for Persons with Multiple Sclerosis. In C. F. Waltz & O. L. Strickland (Eds.), *Measurement of nursing outcomes: Vol. 1: Measuring client centered outcomes* (pp. 128–159.) New York: Springer Publishing Co.

Gulick, E. E. (1988b). Concurrent validity for the ADL Self-Care Scale. *Proceedings of the national symposium of nursing research,* Promoting quality of patient care through research, pp. 91–95. San Francisco, CA.

Gulick, E. E. (1991a). Self-assessed health and use of health services. *Western Journal of Nursing Research, 13,* 195–219.

Gulick E. E. (1991b). Reliability and validity of the Work Assessment Scale for Persons with Multiple Sclerosis. *Nursing Research, 40,* 107–112.

Gulick, E. E. (1992). Model for predicting work performance among persons with multiple sclerosis. *Nursing Research, 41,* 266–272.

Gulick, E. E. (1994). Social support among persons with multiple sclerosis. *Research in Nursing & Health, 17,* 195–206.

Gulick, E. E. (1995). Coping among spouses or significant others of persons with multiple sclerosis. *Nursing Research, 44,* 220–225.

Gulick, E. E. (1996). Health status, work impediments, and coping related to work roles of women with multiple sclerosis. *WORK, A Journal of Prevention, Assessment and Rehabilitation, 6,* 153–166.

Gulick, E. E. (1997). Correlates of quality of life among persons with multiple sclerosis. *Nursing Research, 46,* 305–311.

Gulick, E. E. (1998). Symptom and activities of daily living trajectory in multiple sclerosis: A 10–year study. *Nursing Research, 47,* 137–146.

Gulick, E. E. (2001). Emotional distress and activities of daily living functioning in persons with multiple sclerosis. *Nursing Research, 50,* 117 154.

Gulick, E. E., & Bugg, A. (1992). Holistic health patterning in multiple sclerosis. *Research in Nursing & Health, 15,* 175–185.

Gulick, E. E., Cook, S. D., & Troiano, R. (1993). Comparison of patient and staff assessment of MS patients' health status. *Acta Neurologica Scandinavica, 88,* 87–93.

International Federation of Multiple Sclerosis Societies. (1985). *Minimum record of disability in multiple sclerosis.* New York: National Multiple Sclerosis Society.

Jeffreys, M., Millard, J. M., Human, M., & Warren, M. D. (1969). A set of tests for measuring motor impairment in prevalence studies. *Journal of Chronic Diseases, 22,* 303–319.

Kaufert, J. M. (1983). Functional ability indices: Measurement problems in assessing their validity. *Archives of Physical Medicine and Rehabilitation, 64,* 260–267.

Keith, R. A. (1984). Functional assessment measures in medical rehabilitation current status. *Archives of Physical Medicine and Rehabilitation, 65,* 74–78.

McCorkle, R., & Benoliel, J. Q. (1981). *Cancer patient responses to psychosocial variables.* Seattle, WA: University of Washington, Community Health Care Systems Department.

Orem, D. E. (1980). *Nursing: Concepts of practice* (2nd ed.). New York: McGraw-Hill.

Orem, D. E. (1991). *Nursing: Concepts of practice* (4ᵗʰ ed.). New York: McGraw-Hill.

Robinson-Smith, G. (1993). Coping and life satisfaction after stroke. *Journal of Cerebrovascular Diseases, 3,* 209–215.

Vickrey, B. G., Hays, R. D., Genovese, B. J., Myers, L. W., & Ellison, G. W. (1997). Comparison of a generic to disease-targeted health-related quality-of-life measures for multiple sclerosis. *Journal of Clinical Epidemiology, 50,* 557–569.

Wineman, N. M., Durand, E. J., & Steiner, R. P. (1994). A comparative analysis of coping behaviors in persons with multiple sclerosis or a spinal cord injury. *Research in Nursing and Health, 17,* 185–194.

APPENDIX
Short Form

ADL SELF-CARE SCALE©

ID: _____
Date: _____

Scale completed by:

___ Person with MS
___ Spouse/Partner
___ Relative/Friend
___ Other, describe

Directions:

Fifteen statements about activities of daily living (ADL) such as dressing, walking, and travel are presented. Please rate each statement according to how frequently **YOU** perform the behavior. Base your ratings on a **TYPICAL** day. On the next page you are asked to rate 12 of the questions again according to how much **HELP FROM OTHERS** you receive in performing each activity. Thank you.

Check (✔) how frequently **YOU DO** the following activities on a **typical day.**	Never 0	Almost Never 1	Occasionally 2	Usually 3	Almost Always 4	Always 5
Cut your food						
Get in and out of the tub or shower						
Turn from side to side while in a lying position						
Work buttons/zippers/laces						
Walk inside the house						
Walk up or down a ramp						
Get to and from your present method of travel (car, bus, etc)						
Read printed material						
Use a telephone						
Write clearly						
Participate in social activities outside the home						
Participate in recreational activities outside the home						
Confide in someone special						
Exchange loving glances with someone special						
Experience satisfactory sexual activity						

©Gulick (1987).

ADL SCALE: HELP FROM OTHERS©

Check (✔) how frequently YOU need HELP FROM OTHERS to do the following activities on a **typical day.**	Never 0	Almost Never 1	Occas- sionally 2	Usually 3	Almost Always 4	Always 5
Cut your food						
Get in and out of the tub or shower						
Turn from side to side while in a lying position						
Work buttons/zippers/laces						
Walk inside the house						
Walk up or down a ramp						
Get to and from your present method of travel (car, bus, etc)						
Read printed material						
Use a telephone						
Write clearly						
Participate in social activities outside the home						
Participate in recreational activities outside the home						

©Gulick (1987).

LONG FORM

ADL SELF-CARE SCALE©

Scale completed by:

_____ Person with MS
_____ Spouse/Partner
_____ Relative/Friend
_____ Other, describe

ID: _____
Date: _____

Directions:
Eleven activities of daily living (ADL) such as dressing, walking, toileting and so forth are each described by five statements. Please rate each statement according to **WHAT YOU PRESENTLY DO.** Base your ratings on a **TYPICAL** day. You will then be asked to rate ten of these activities again according to how much **HELP FROM OTHERS** you receive in performing each activity.

Rate each activity according to what you do on a **TYPICAL** day. The ratings include:

Never	Almost Never	Occasionally	Usually	Almost Always	Always
0	1	2	3	4	5

A Self-Care ADL Profile with instructions is attached for persons who wish to plot their own functional level among the 11 activities.

Thank you.

1. EATING

Self-Care

Check (✔) how frequently **YOU DO** the following activities on a **typical day.**	Never 0	Almost Never 1	Occas-sionally 2	Usually 3	Almost Always 4	Always 5
Prepare meals and/or transfer food from one place to another						
Cut your food						
Pour liquids						
Open milk cartons or similar containers						
Feed yourself						

©Gulick 1987.

Help from Others

Check (✔) how frequently **YOU** need **HELP FROM OTHERS** to do the following activities on a **typical day.**	Never 0	Almost Never 1	Occas-sionally 2	Usually 3	Almost Always 4	Always 5
Prepare meals and/or transfer food from one place to another						
Cut your food						
Pour liquids						
Open milk cartons or similar containers						
Feed yourself						

2. DRESSING

Self-Care

Check (✔) how frequently **YOU DO** the following activities on a **typical day.**

	Never 0	Almost Never 1	Occas- sionally 2	Usually 3	Almost Always 4	Always 5
Put on underwear						
Put on socks/stockings/shoes/braces						
Work buttons/zippers/laces						
Put on trousers/dresses, shirts, coats, or other items						
Remove your own clothes						

Help from Others

Check (✔) how frequently **YOU** need **HELP FROM OTHERS** to do the following activities on a **typical day.**

	Never 0	Almost Never 1	Occas- sionally 2	Usually 3	Almost Always 4	Always 5
Put on underwear						
Put on socks/stockings/shoes/braces						
Work buttons/zippers/laces						
Put on trousers/dresses, shirts, coats, or other items						
Remove your own clothes						

3. WALKING

Self-Care

Check (✔) how frequently **YOU DO** the following activities on a **typical day.**	Never 0	Almost Never 1	Occas-sionally 2	Usually 3	Almost Always 4	Always 5
Walk inside the house						
Walk outside the house (minimum of one block)						
Walk on uneven ground surfaces						
Walk up or down a ramp						
Climb and walk down one flight of stairs						

Help from Others

Check (✔) how frequently **YOU** need **HELP FROM OTHERS** to do the following activities on a **typical day.**	Never 0	Almost Never 1	Occas-sionally 2	Usually 3	Almost Always 4	Always 5
Walk inside the house						
Walk outside the house (minimum of one block)						
Walk on uneven ground surfaces						
Walk up or down a ramp						
Climb and walk down one flight of stairs						

4. TRANSFER

Self-Care

Check (✔) how frequently **YOU DO** the following activities on a **typical day.**	Never 0	Almost Never 1	Occas- sionally 2	Usually 3	Almost Always 4	Always 5
Turn from side to side while in a lying position						
Get into a sitting position from lying and vice versa						
Get from sitting to standing and vice versa						
Get from one sitting position to another sitting position						
Transfer only with assistance of mechanical devices such as a patient lift						

Help from Others

Check (✔) how frequently **YOU** need **HELP FROM OTHERS** to do the following activities on a **typical day.**	Never 0	Almost Never 1	Occas- sionally 2	Usually 3	Almost Always 4	Always 5
Turn from side to side while in a lying position						
Get into a sitting position from lying and vice versa						
Get from sitting to standing and vice versa						
Get from one sitting position to another sitting position						
Transfer only with assistance of mechanical devices such as a patient lift						

147

5. TRAVEL

Check (✔) the type of travel you use most frequently:

___ Car ___ bus ___ train ___ airplane ___ wheelchair ___ other, describe _____

Self-Care

Check (✔) how frequently YOU DO the following activities on a **typical day.**	Never 0	Almost Never 1	Occas- sionally 2	Usually 3	Almost Always 4	Always 5
Get to and from your present method of travel (car, bus, other)						
Get on and off your present method of travel (car, bus, other)						
Get into, through, and out of buildings						
Travel long distances						
Travel freely as desired						

Help from Others

Check (✔) how frequently YOU need **HELP FROM OTHERS** to do the following activities on a **typical day.**	Never 0	Almost Never 1	Occas- sionally 2	Usually 3	Almost Always 4	Always 5
Get to and from your present method of travel (car, bus, other)						
Get on and off your present method of travel (car, bus, other)						
Get into, through, and out of buildings						
Travel long distances						
Travel freely as desired						

6. BATHING

Self-Care

Check (✔) how frequently YOU **DO** the following activities on a **typical day.**	Never 0	Almost Never 1	Occas- sionally 2	Usually 3	Almost Always 4	Always 5
Get in and out of the bathroom						
Get in and out of the tub or shower						
Get water and bath supplies						
Wash "hard to reach" body parts						
Wash all body parts (total bath)						

Help from Others

Check (✔) how frequently YOU need **HELP FROM OTHERS** to do the following activities on a **typical day.**	Never 0	Almost Never 1	Occas- sionally 2	Usually 3	Almost Always 4	Always 5
Get in and out of the bathroom						
Get in and out of the tub or shower						
Get water and bath supplies						
Wash "hard to reach" body parts						
Wash all body parts (total bath)						

7. TOILETING—URINATION

Self-Care

Check (✔) how frequently **YOU DO** the following activities on a **typical day.**	Never 0	Almost Never 1	Occas-sionally 2	Usually 3	Almost Always 4	Always 5
Limit the amount of fluid you drink to control urine accidents						
Take medication to control urine problems						
Apply hand pressure over the bladder to assist with bladder emptying						
Use an absorbent pad or external catheter or sheath because of urine leakage						
Perform intermittent self-catheterization						

Help from Others

Check (✔) how frequently **YOU** need **HELP FROM OTHERS** to do the following activities on a **typical day.**	Never 0	Almost Never 1	Occas-sionally 2	Usually 3	Almost Always 4	Always 5
Limit the amount of fluid you drink to control urine accidents						
Take medication to control urine problems						
Apply hand pressure over the bladder to assist with bladder emptying						
Use an absorbent pad or external catheter or sheath because of urine leakage						
Perform intermittent self-catheterization						

8. TOILETING—BOWEL

Self-Care

Check (✔) how frequently **YOU DO** the following activities on a **typical day.**	Never 0	Almost Never 1	Occas- sionally 2	Usually 3	Almost Always 4	Always 5
Use special foods to promote normal bowel movements						
Use laxatives or other medicines						
Use suppositories						
Use enemas						
Wear a diaper						

Help from Others

Check (✔) how frequently **YOU** need **HELP FROM OTHERS** to do the following activities on a **typical day.**	Never 0	Almost Never 1	Occas- sionally 2	Usually 3	Almost Always 4	Always 5
Use special foods to promote normal bowel movements						
Use laxatives or other medicines						
Use suppositories						
Use enemas						
Wear a diaper						

9. RECREATION AND SOCIALIZING

Self-Care

Check (✔) how frequently **YOU DO** the following activities on a **typical day.**	Never 0	Almost Never 1	Occas- sionally 2	Usually 3	Almost Always 4	Always 5
Participate in social activities outside the home						
Participate socially with visitors in the home						
Participate socially with family members in the home						
Participate in recreational activities outside the home						
Participate in recreational activities inside the home						

Help from Others

Check (✔) how frequently **YOU** need **HELP FROM OTHERS** to do the following activities on a **typical day.**	Never 0	Almost Never 1	Occas- sionally 2	Usually 3	Almost Always 4	Always 5
Participate in social activities outside the home						
Participate socially with visitors in the home						
Participate socially with family members in the home						
Participate in recreational activities outside the home						
Participate in recreational activities inside the home						

10. SENSORY AND COMMUNICATION

Self-Care

Check (✔) how frequently YOU DO the following activities on a **typical day.**	Never 0	Almost Never 1	Occas- sionally 2	Usually 3	Almost Always 4	Always 5
Read printed or written material						
Hear what other persons are saying at normal speaking tones						
Speak so other persons can easily understand what you say						
Use a telephone						
Write clearly						

Help from Others

Check (✔) how frequently YOU need HELP FROM OTHERS to do the following activities on a **typical day.**	Never 0	Almost Never 1	Occas- sionally 2	Usually 3	Almost Always 4	Always 5
Read printed or written material						
Hear what other persons are saying at normal speaking tones						
Speak so other persons can easily understand what you say						
Use a telephone						
Write clearly						

11. INTIMACY

Self-Care

Check (✔) how frequently YOU DO the following activities on a **typical day.**	Never 0	Almost Never 1	Occas- sionally 2	Usually 3	Almost Always 4	Almost Always 5
Confide in someone regarding personal matters						
Exchange loving glances with someone special						
Exchange tender touches with someone special						
Share intimate conversations with someone special						
Experience satisfactory sexual activities with someone special						

MS SELF-CARE ADL PROFILE

Directions for completing your ADL PROFILE

1. Sum the 5 ratings for the **SELF-CARE** and **HELP FROM OTHERS** scales
2. Place an (0) on the graph below that corresponds to the activity and rating score obtained for **SELF-CARE**
3. Place an (X) on the graph below that corresponds to the activity and rating score obtained for **HELP FROM OTHERS**
4. Draw a blue line to connect the 0's and draw a red line to connect the X's.
5. Subtract the **HELP FROM OTHERS** score from the **SELF-CARE** score and record the difference score below each respective activity. A positive score suggests greater independence in performing ADL and a negative score suggests greater dependency on other persons to perform those activities.

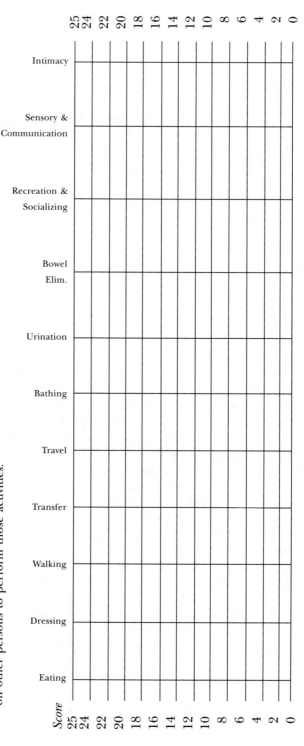

Difference Score: _ _ _ _ _ _ _ _ _ _ _ _

155

10

The Touch Instrument

Alicia Huckstadt

This chapter discusses the Touch Instrument, a measure of the responses of the recipient to touch.

PURPOSE

In health care interactions touch is a frequent intervention that is used for a variety of reasons. Touch is a means of communicating caring, support, and empathy; establishing rapport; and giving physical care. Unfortunately, touch may be misinterpreted, and the effect of the touch is often not known. The Touch Instrument provides nurses and other health care providers with an instrument that includes an assessment of the touch given, specific physiological and psychological responses, and the effects of the touch as perceived by the recipient. More specifically, the purpose of the Touch Instrument is to assess the characteristics of the touch, the toucher, and the recipient of touch (Part I); to measure the physiological and psychological changes occurring during and after the recipient is touched (Part II); and to measure the perceived effects by the recipient of the touch (Part III).

The objectives of the measure are as follows:

1. to obtain pertinent demographic information on the toucher and the recipient of the touch
2. to assess the type and other characteristics of the touch given to the recipient
3. to assess physiological and psychological measures before, during, and after the touch
4. to assess the recipient's perception of the effect of the touch

CONCEPTUAL BASIS OF THE TOUCH INSTRUMENT

Touch is conceptually defined as a sensory system that provides physiological, psychological, and social effects for the toucher and the recipient. Its initiation and interpretation are determined by numerous factors, such as the toucher's and recipient's age, gender, self-esteem, culture; relationship between individuals involved; reciprocity; body parts involved; setting and circumstances; and the type, quality, duration, intensity, temperature, and location of the touch (Huckstadt, 1990). In nursing, touch is primarily viewed as a communicative technique (often called expressive or supportive touch) or as a means of assessing, monitoring, and providing physical care (often called procedural, technical, or instrumental touch). Weiss (1986) reported that nurses need to be conscious of their touch given to patients. Although studies have demonstrated the positive effects of touch by health providers, some touch may produce negative physiological and psychological effects in patients such as increased nervous system arousal. Weiss (1979) discussed the conceptual framework of touch in nursing research and practice. Using neurological and sociopsychological theory and research, Weiss described the six major tactile symbols in the language of touch: (1) duration—temporal length of touch; (2) location—area of the body contacted, including threshold, extent, and centripetality; (3) action or rate of approach to a body surface with the attendant amount of physical energy exerted in the onset of the touch; (4) intensity—extent of indentation applied to the body surface by the pressure of the touch; (5) frequency—amount of touching; and (6) sensation—reaction to the touch. The significance of these symbols lies in their power to affect an individual's perception ability for sensory discrimination of his or her body, the pleasure/pain balance of the body, and self-cathexis, specifically for approval or liking of one's body.

Weiss indicated that an assessment of the tactile environment, including the nurse's own determination of the purpose of the touch and the patient's tactile response disposition, is an important consideration of patient care. The therapeutic nature of the touch will be dependent on the congruency between the nurse and the patient within the tactile environment.

Some attempt has been made to categorize touch in health professions. Watson (1975) identified two types of touching by personnel (nurse, nurse's aide, orderly) in a geriatric nursing home. Instrumental touch was identified as the intentional physical contact occurring when another task is being performed, and expressive touch was identified as the touch that does not require a task component and is spontaneous and affective (e.g., comforting a patient).

PROCEDURES FOR DEVELOPMENT

Using pertinent literature, the Touch Instrument incorporated those items believed to influence touch and how the touch is perceived by the toucher and the recipient. The recipient's perceptions include those factors identified in the literature that are thought to be positive and negative outcomes of touch, including some items from previous work by Stolte (1976). Items were designed to address each of the objectives of the instrument. Therefore, sections were included that addressed the description of the touch given, the description of the toucher, the nature and location of the touch, the effect of the touch, and the patient's emotional response or perception of the touch.

DESCRIPTION

The Touch Instrument was developed in a checklist and questionnaire format and has three distinct parts. Part I is "Description of Touch Given," and collects descriptive information on the toucher, recipient, and the nature of the touch. Part II is "Effect of Touch," and assesses the physiological and psychological response to touch. Part III is "Patient's Perception," and is a semantic differential scale with 31 opposite adjective pairs or descriptors of the patient's feelings and perceptions upon being touched. Each item in Part III provides for a seven-step response from 1 through 7. The Touch Instrument will be found in the Appendix to this chapter.

ADMINISTRATION AND SCORING

Parts I and II may be completed by the toucher or an observer (the demographic data, and items 28, 29, and 30 of Part I require the toucher's self-report). Items 7 through 14 of Part I may be obtained by interview and from information in the patient's medical record. Part III is a questionnaire to be given to the recipient of the touch (preferably by someone other than the toucher).

Part I takes approximately 5 to 10 minutes to complete; Part II will vary in time, depending on when physiological and psychological effects are measured; and Part III may take the recipient approximately 10 minutes to complete.

The Touch Instrument is scored as follows: Part I is not scored but provides a description of the toucher, the recipient, and the touch given. Part II is scored by starting with the total number of physiological items being measured (e.g., three items). All items that are not included in the assessment should be designated by NA (not applicable). For every item that changed toward a more relaxed state, a 3 is recorded; for every item that did not change in either direction (stayed the same), a 2 is recorded; for every item that changed toward a tensed state, a 1 is recorded. The points are then summed (range of points from 3 to 9, if three items are evaluated) for each subject. A percentage score can be calculated by comparing the points recorded to the total number of possible points. The same scoring procedure applies to the psychological section. The higher the total score and percentage score for each of the two sections, the more positive the physiological and psychological reaction to the touch. The lapsed time after touch will be recorded without any additional scoring. Part III contains a semantic-differential scale with steps numbered 1 to 7 (1 depicting the most positive state). Subjects indicate how they feel about the touch they received by selecting a number on the scale for each of the 31 items. Items 2, 5, 7, 8, 9, 11, 13, 18, 22, 24, 27, 30 are scored in reverse order. The subject's responses are summed for a total number. The range of possible scores is 31 to 217. The lower the score, the more positive the perception of the touch received. Items 32, 33, and 34 are not scored but provide further information about the recipient of the touch.

RELIABILITY AND VALIDITY EVIDENCE

Reliability

The Touch Instrument is intended to measure a state attribute. Therefore, it was not expected that a stability procedure (test-retest) would yield a high correlation in nurse–patient interactions unless replicated simulations were used. A test–retest correlation was determined in simulated situations in which 15 nursing students received the same audiovisual situations. A Pearson product moment correlation coefficient of .82 for scores on Part III was obtained from test to retest with a two–week interval for a procedural touch simulation and a Pearson's correlation coefficient of .76 for a supportive touch simulation.

Interrater reliability was assessed for Parts I and II. Two master's prepared nurses viewed the same nurse–patient interaction, which included a report of the physiological values for the patient. A 91% agreement was obtained for all items.

Internal consistency was assessed for Part III using Cronbach's alpha. Alpha coefficients ranging from .81 to .97 were obtained for the study, which used simulated nurse–patient supportive and procedural touch interactions. In a study of 41 adult hospitalized patients an alpha coefficient of .97 was found. Internal consistency for Part II (physiological) revealed an alpha of .45. The alpha for the psychological section of Part II could not be computed due to zero variance. An additional study of five rural hospitalized patients revealed an internal consistency alpha of 0.95. The item-to-total correlations for the 31 items in Part III for both groups of hospitalized patients (N = 46) ranged from .40 to .87.

Validity

Content validity was determined for each part through review of the literature and review by three nurse researchers in the area of touch. Two judges evaluated the relevancy of each item, and a content validity index of 0.88 was obtained. The third judge provided written support for the instrument.

Construct validity was evaluated using a contrasted-groups approach within a simulated setting. Seventeen nursing students were provided with two audiovisual situations in which the 17 subjects, in the role of patients, responded to items on Part III of the instrument. The first situation included supportive touch provided by a nurse to a patient; the second situation included a painful procedural touch by a nurse to a patient. Paired-samples t tests revealed significant differences for responses to the two types of touch (df = 16, t = −10.56, p = .0001). The simulations were repeated two weeks later with the same subjects, and significant differences were again found (df = 16, t = −14.16, p = .0001).

Construct validity was also assessed, using a group of 41 hospitalized adult patients who were randomly assigned to an experimental group or control group. The experimental group received two to five minutes of supportive touch in a patient–nurse interaction during routine care. The control group received a verbal interaction without any touch. Blood pressure, respiration, and pulse were monitored and a brief psychological assessment was conducted before and after the interactions. Patients were then requested to complete Part III, including a one-item patient-satisfaction visual analogue scale (Item 34); t-tests for independent samples revealed significant differences between the experimental and control groups in their responses to Items 1 through 31 of Part III (df = 39, t = −2.95, p = .005) and patient satisfaction scores (df = 39, t = 2.17, p = .036). Although subjects in the touch group had more positive physiological assessment scores, there were no significant differences between groups for physiological or psychological assessment scores (Part II).

Concurrent validity was assessed by correlating Part III scores with the patient visual analogue item (34). Pearson's correlation coefficients were calculated for the nursing students' (N = 15) simulated nurse–patient interactions: −.79, p = .0001, for patient satisfaction and supportive touch and −.61, p = .008, for patient satisfaction and procedural touch.

CONCLUSIONS AND RECOMMENDATIONS

The Touch Instrument includes a comprehensive assessment of touch and items that measure the physiological, psychological, and perceived effects of the touch by the recipient. Further refinement of the instrument is needed. The low alpha levels relating to Part II and the insignificant difference between the hospitalized patient groups (touch and no touch) suggest a need to examine better ways to measure the physiological effects of touch. Another concern relates to social desirability, which may possibly confound subject perception scores. Efforts were made in this psychometric study to assure patients that their responses were not going to be used in any manner other than for the development of the instrument. In addition, they were assured that there were no right or wrong responses. It is suggested that a measure of social desirability be included in future work, however.

ACKNOWLEDGMENT

This study was partially funded by The Wichita State University, School of Nursing. The assistance of expert panel members, Ruth McCorkle, RN, PhD, Karen Stolte, RN, PhD, and Sandra Weiss, RN, PhD, as well as the assistance of Bonnie Krenning, RN, MSN; Mary Koehn, RN, MSN; and Maurice Tinterow, MD, PhD (deceased), is acknowledged.

REFERENCES

Huckstadt, A. (1990). The Touch Instrument. In O. L. Strickland & C. F. Waltz, *Measurement of nursing outcomes: Vol. 4: Measuring client self-care and coping skills* (pp. 267–285). New York: Springer Publishing Co.

Stolte, K. M. (1976). *An exploratory study of patients' perceptions of the touch they received during labor.* Unpublished doctoral dissertation, University of Kansas, Lawrence.

Watson, W. H. (1975). The meaning of touch: Geriatric nursing. *Journal of Communication, 25,* 104–112.

Weiss, S. J. (1979). The language of touch. *Nursing Research, 28,* 76–80.

Weiss, S. J. (1986). Psychophysiological effects of caregiver touch on incidence of cardiac dysrhythmia. *Heart and Lung, 15,* 495–505.

APPENDIX: THE TOUCH INSTRUMENT

Part I. Description of Touch Given

Directions: Please place a checkmark in the space to the left of your response and fill in the blanks as indicated.

TOUCHER   RECIPIENT

1. Sex:___M ____ F   7. Sex: ____M ____F
2. Age: ____   8. Age: ____
3. Marital Status: 9. Marital Status:
   ____ Single   ____ Single
   ____ Married   ____ Married
   ____ Widowed   ____ Widowed
   ____ Divorced   ____ Divorced
4. Ethnic Group: 10. Ethnic Group:
   ____ Asian   ____ Asian
   ____ White   ____ White
   ____ Black   ____ Black
   ____ American Indian   ____ American Indian
   ____ Hispanic   ____ Hispanic
   ____ Other, specify   ____ Other, specify
5. Highest Education Level: 11. Highest Education Level:
   ____ Less than 12 years   ____ Less than 12 years
   ____ High School graduate   ____ High School graduate
   ____ Diploma in Nursing   ____ Some college, no degree
   ____ Some college, no degree   ____ Associate degree
   ____ Associate degree   ____ Baccalaureate degree
   ____ Baccalaureate degree   ____ Masters degree
   ____ Masters degree   ____ Doctoral degree
   ____ Doctoral degree
6. Status of Toucher: 12. Medical Diagnosis:
   ____ Family member, specify
   relationship_____
   _____
   ____ Friend
   ____ Student Nurse   13. Existing Sensory Problems
   ____ R.N.   _____
   ____ L.P.N.   _____
   ____ Aide or Orderly
   ____ Physician   14. Current Medications
   ____ Other _____   Affecting Sensorium:
                                      _____

COMPLETE FOR EACH TOUCH GIVEN:

15. Setting in which Touch Occurred
    ____ Recipient's room
    ____ Recipient's bathroom
    ____ Hallway
    ____ Dining room
    ____Other, describe _____

16. Type of Touch Given
    ____ Technical (involving a procedure), describe _____
    _____
    ____ Expressive (comforting), describe _____
    _____

17. Source of Touch Given (What touched the recipient?)
    ____ Hand ____ Arm ____ Shoulder
    ____ Other, describe_____

18. Location of Touch Given—mark location with an X on the body
    figure below. Both a front view and a back view are pictured.

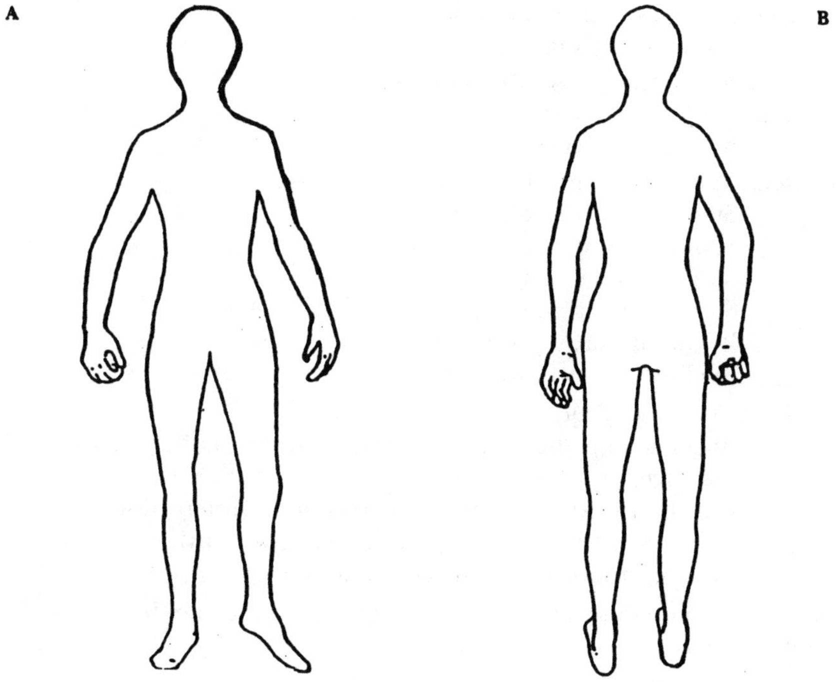

FIGURE 10.1. Body figure. **A:** Front view; **B:** back view.

19. Duration of Touch Given
    ____ Less than 1 second
    ____ 1 second to 15 seconds
    ____ 16 seconds to 60 seconds
    ____ 61 seconds to 2 minutes
    ____ More than 2 minutes, approximate time

20. Initial Intensity of Touch Given
    ____ No indentation
    ____ Slight indentation
    ____ Moderate indentation
    ____ Strong indentation

21. Intensity Variation of Touch Given
    ____ No indentation
    ____ Slight indentation
    ____ Moderate indentation
    ____ Strong indentation

22. Action (specific gesture or movement) of the Touch
    ____ Stroke
    ____ Pat
    ____ Grasp, Squeeze
    ____ Other, specify _____

23. Toucher's Position When Touch was Given
    ____ Standing, facing recipient
    ____ Standing, not facing recipient
    ____ Sitting, facing recipient
    ____ Sitting, not facing recipient

24. Recipient's Position When Touch Was Given
    ____ Standing, facing toucher
    ____ Standing, not facing toucher
    ____ Sitting, facing toucher
    ____ Sitting, not facing toucher
    ____ Reclining, facing toucher
    ____ Reclining, not facing toucher

25. When Was the Touch Given?
    ____ Approaching the recipient (occurs when first interacting with
         the recipient)
    ____ Interfacing with the recipient (occurs as interaction stabilizes)
    ____ Separating from the recipient (occurs as individual prepares to
         end the interaction and leave the area)

26. Other Communication Channels Accompanying the Touch Used by
    the Toucher
    ____ Eye contact
    ____ Verbal

____ Smiling
____ Frowning
____ Other body/facial gestures, describe _____
_____

27. How was the Touch Reciprocated by the Recipient?
____ Was not reciprocated
____ Touch was returned, describe type and location _____
_____

____ Verbal expression. What was said? _____
_____

____ Turned head toward toucher
____ Turned body toward toucher
____ Made direct eye contact
____ Smiling
____ Frowning
____ Other body/facial gestures, describe _____
_____

The following items (23, 29, 30) require the response of the Toucher

28. What was the intended action of the touch? _____
_____

29. What was the expected sensation for the recipient of the touch? _____
_____

30. Did the toucher feel comfortable touching?
____ Yes
____ No

31. Additional Comments

Part II. Effect of Touch

Directions: Record the before touch measurement, the during touch measurement (if patient has a continuous monitor), the after touch measurement, and the length of lapsed time since touch was given.

	Before Touch	During Touch	After Touch	Lapsed Time After Touch
Physiological:				
1. Blood Pressure	_____	_____	_____	_____
2. Pulse Rate	_____	_____	_____	_____
3. Respiratory Rate	_____	_____	_____	_____
4. Other, specify				
_____	_____	_____	_____	_____

Psychological:

5. Orientation	___ Alert	___ Alert	___ Alert
	___ Confused	___ Confused	___ Confused
6. Willingness to cooperate	___ Yes	___ Yes	___ Yes
	___ No	___ No	___ No
7. Willingness to self-disclose	___ Yes	___ Yes	___ Yes
	___ No	___ No	___ No
8. Other, specify			

12. Additional Comments:

Part III. Patient's Perception

Directions: There are many feelings that we have when someone inter-acts with us. Please read each of the following items and place a check mark on the line of each item to describe how you felt about the interaction you have just had with the nurse. For example, on the Cared or/Neglected word pair, 1 = totally cared for; 2 = moderately cared for; 3 = slightly cared for; 4 = neutral; 5 = slightly neglected; 6 = moderately neglected; 7 = totally neglected. There are no right or wrong responses.

The interaction made me feel:

[*Editorial Note: Descriptors as noted above should be placed vertically above each number it represents at the top of the scale below.*]

1. Cared for	___:___:___:___:___:___:___ 1 2 3 4 5 6 7	Neglected
2. Upset	___:___:___:___:___:___:___ 1 2 3 4 5 6 7	Reassured
3. Comfortable	___:___:___:___:___:___:___ 1 2 3 4 5 6 7	Uncomfortable
4. Worthy	___:___:___:___:___:___:___ 1 2 3 4 5 6 7	Unworthy
5. Unhappy	___:___:___:___:___:___:___ 1 2 3 4 5 6 7	Happy

6. Courageous   __:__:__:__:__:__:__   Scared
              1   2   3   4   5   6   7

7. Unaccepted   __:__:__:__:__:__:__   Accepted
              1   2   3   4   5   6   7

8. Distrustful   __:__:__:__:__:__:__   Trustful
              1   2   3   4   5   6   7

9. Physically tense   __:__:__:__:__:__:__   Physically relaxed
              1   2   3   4   5   6   7

10. Good   __:__:__:__:__:__:__   Bad
              1   2   3   4   5   6   7

11. Unsure   __:__:__:__:__:__:__   Confident
              1   2   3   4   5   6   7

12. Helped   __:__:__:__:__:__:__   Not helped
              1   2   3   4   5   6   7

13. More pain   __:__:__:__:__:__:__   Less pain
              1   2   3   4   5   6   7

14. Less anxious   __:__:__:__:__:__:__   More anxious
              1   2   3   4   5   6   7

15. Pleasant   __:__:__:__:__:__:__   Unpleasant
              1   2   3   4   5   6   7

16. Better   __:__:__:__:__:__:__   Worse
              1   2   3   4   5   6   7

17. Secure   __:__:__:__:__:__:__   Threatened
              1   2   3   4   5   6   7

18. Uncooperative   __:__:__:__:__:__:__   Cooperative
              1   2   3   4   5   6   7

19. Willing to share feelings   __:__:__:__:__:__:__   Unwilling to share feelings
              1   2   3   4   5   6   7

20. Understood   __:__:__:__:__:__:__   Misunderstood
              1   2   3   4   5   6   7

21. Closer to the nurse   __:__:__:__:__:__:__   More distant
              1   2   3   4   5   6   7

22. Alone   __:__:__:__:__:__:__   Supported
              1   2   3   4   5   6   7

23. Safe   __:__:__:__:__:__:__   Unsafe
              1   2   3   4   5   6   7

24. Less aware   __:__:__:__:__:__:__   More aware
              1   2   3   4   5   6   7

25. Respected   __:__:__:__:__:__:__   Ignored
              1   2   3   4   5   6   7

26. Calm   ___:___:___:___:___:___:___   Annoyed
               1   2   3   4   5   6   7

27. Discouraged   ___:___:___:___:___:___:___   Encouraged
               1   2   3   4   5   6   7

28. Warm   ___:___:___:___:___:___:___   Cold
               1   2   3   4   5   6   7

29. Restful   ___:___:___:___:___:___:___   Restless
               1   2   3   4   5   6   7

30. Less able to do   ___:___:___:___:___:___:___   More able to do
               1   2   3   4   5   6   7

31. More aware of   ___:___:___:___:___:___:___   Less aware of
    what person was   1   2   3   4   5   6   7   what person
    saying   was saying

Directions: Please answer the following questions by placing a check-mark in the space preceding your response to each item.

32. Would you consider yourself a
    ____toucher (I like to touch or be touched by other people)
    ____nontoucher (I do not like to touch or be touched by others)

33. How many times have you been hospitalized?
    _____ None
    _____1 time
    _____2 times
    _____3 times
    _____4 times
    _____5 or more times

34. *Directions:* Please place an X on the line below indicating how satisfied you are with the care you are receiving at the current time.
    Very satisfied _____Very dissatisfied

THANK YOU FOR YOUR PARTICIPATION.

11

Measuring Attentional Demands in Community-Dwelling Elders

Debra A. Jansen and Mary L. Keller

This chapter discusses the Attentional Demands Survey, a measure of attentional demands of community-dwelling elders.

PURPOSE

In day-to-day life, people rely on a pivotal facet of cognitive functioning, the capacity to direct attention (CDA). CDA allows people to effectively manage daily tasks, particularly those requiring one to process complex information, make decisions, and acquire new skills. Loss of CDA has been shown to interfere with intellectual and reflective skills (Lezak, 1995; Mesulam, 1985), heighten the risk for falling and driving accidents (Brown, Shumway-Cook, & Woollacott, 1999; McKnight & McKnight, 1999), and impair social functioning (Tun, 1998; van Zomeren, & Brouwer, 1994). As people age, CDA appears to decline (Cimprich, 1993a, 1998; Jansen, 1997; McDowd & Shaw, 2000; Parasuraman & Greenwood, 1998). Two reasons have been proposed: 1) aging is associated with unique and growing demands on attentional mechanisms, including those created by difficulties with hearing, vision, and mobility; and (2) physiological changes in the brain with age may reduce baseline levels of CDA. As a result, older people face considerable attentional demands and fewer attentional resources to manage them (Jansen & Keller, 1998). The purpose of this chapter is to describe the theoretical basis and the psychometric development of a tool to measure the attentional demands of community-dwelling elders. It may be possible for nurses to assist elders to conserve attentional resources by designing interventions that reduce attentional demands. An important step in this line of research is the development of an instrument to measure attentional demands.

CONCEPTUAL BASIS OF THE ATTENTIONAL DEMANDS SURVEY

An evolving theoretical framework of directed attentional fatigue and restoration by Kaplan and Kaplan (1983, 1989; Kaplan, 1995) was the basis for the development of the Attentional Demands Survey. Cimprich (1992a, 1992b, 1993b, 1995, 1998) has been further developing the framework in her work with women recovering from breast cancer. Central concepts include the capacity to direct attention (CDA), attentional demands, directed attentional fatigue (DAF), restoration, and neurological influences (Figure 11.1).

CDA is a type of selective attention. It involves the use of neural inhibitory mechanisms to focus the mind on the meaningful aspects of a situation and block out distractions and less relevant information. However, sustained use of CDA for prolonged periods of time is mentally effortful, implying the necessity of resting this capacity (Kaplan, 1995). Attentional demands are factors that increase the need for directed attention. They serve as distracting and competing stimuli that must be inhibited if people are to maintain focus and achieve mental clarity. The presence of attentional demands requires intensive use of CDA, and thus can fatigue the neural inhibitory mechanisms, a condition known as directed atten-

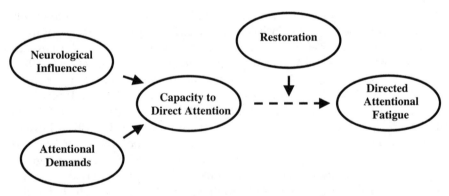

FIGURE 11.1 A proposed model illustrating the theoretical framework. Neurological influences associated with aging physiologically lower Capacity to Direct Attention (CDA). Attentional demands are factors that increase the expenditure of CDA, thereby depleting it. Under the presences of neurological influences and a degree of attentional demands that exceeds the older person's available level of CDA, directed attentional fatigue (DAF) results. However, restoration may buffer the effects of the attentional demands on CDA so that DAF can be prevented or alleviated.
From Jansen & Keller (1999).

tional fatigue (DAF). DAF occurs when a person is exposed to a level of attentional demands that exceeds his or her baseline capacity. It is manifested as a decline in CDA evidenced by difficulty managing everyday tasks; frustration, irritability, and trouble remembering and making decisions; and is objectively demonstrated by poorer performance on attention tests (Cimprich, 1995; Kaplan & Kaplan, 1983). The concept of restoration refers to activities and environments that enhance and maintain CDA and allow the attentional mechanisms to rest and recover. Theoretically, exposure to mentally restorative activities, particularly those involving nature, such as looking through a window, walking in the park, and gardening, may prevent and alleviate DAF (Cimprich, 1993b; Kaplan & Kaplan, 1989). The final concept, neurological influences, includes physiological processes affecting brain structures, thereby potentially altering CDA (Jansen & Keller, 1999). Examples are changes associated with age such as neuronal atrophy and declines in neurotransmitters, neurological and psychological disorders, lack of sleep, and medications that enhance or interfere with concentration (Raz, 2000; Reuter-Lorenz, 2000).

Because the theoretical framework is relatively new, instruments to measure the concepts are under development. Nurses may be particularly interested in attentional demands because they may be amenable to interventions. For this reason, the researchers have focused on the development of an instrument to measure attentional demands.

Theoretically, attentional demands fall within one of four domains: physical-environmental, informational, behavioral, and affective (Cimprich, 1992a, 1992b, 1995; Jansen & Cimprich, 1994; Jansen & Keller, 1998). Physical-environmental demands are factors in the external environment that make it more difficult to complete tasks because attentional capacity must be devoted to minimizing their effects or managing despite them. Examples include harsh weather conditions, bright sunlight and glare, and insufficient living space and clutter. Greater attentional capacity is needed to manage tasks when these demands are present. Informational demands are factors that make the perception and interpretation of information difficult, such as vision and hearing losses and unclear and conflicting means of presenting information. When informational demands are present, considerably more CDA may be needed to interpret and respond to everyday situations. Behavioral demands are factors of a biophysical, societal, or situational nature that interfere with and restrict one's intended activities and wishes. For instance, behaviors may be restricted in the sense of lacking privacy and independence or of not being free to express oneself because a person lacks a partner with whom to communicate (Jansen & Keller, 1998). CDA is necessary to overcome these obstacles and may be needed to suppress behaviors that cannot be acted upon (Wegner, 1989). Affective demands are feelings and worries that preoccupy and distract. In order to carry on with daily tasks, these distractions and preoccupations must be inhibited, a process that is mentally effortful (Bjorklund & Harnishfeger, 1995; von Hippel, Silver, & Lynch, 2000; Wegner, 1989; Wegner & Erber, 1992).

DEVELOPMENT OF THE ATTENTIONAL DEMANDS SURVEY

Because this was a new area of research, an initial qualitative study (Jansen & Keller, 1998; see Table 11.1) was conducted to assist with the development of items for the Attentional Demands Survey (ADS). The purpose of this first study was to identify the universe of attentional demands experienced by older people. Thirty community-dwelling elderly (22 females, 8 males) were interviewed regarding their experiences with attentional demands within each of the physical-environmental, informational, behavioral, and affective domains. As part of the structured interviews, participants were given brief explanations of attentional demands and of each of the four domains and then asked to describe the demands in their everyday lives. Additional general questions encouraged thoughts missed with the domain-specific queries. These questions and the explanations were reviewed by three researchers knowledgeable in the framework and concerns of the elderly. A content analysis, as outlined by McLaughlin and Marascuilo (1990), was conducted to categorize the interview data into the four domains of attentional demands. Then, the themes within each domain were worded into close-ended Likert-type scale items.

This approach resulted in a 92–item questionnaire. The items were reviewed by knowledgeable researchers involved in developing the framework for theoretical soundness and relevance, comprehensiveness, applicability to the elderly, and clarity and conciseness. Additionally, four elderly individuals participated in a pilot test of the instrument in order to provide feedback on its format and clarity. Based on the feedback from the researchers and the pilot test participants, the questionnaire was reduced from 92 to 67 items.

A second study (Jansen & Keller, 1999; Table 11.1) with 197 community-dwelling elderly was conducted to evaluate the construct validity, internal consistency, and test–retest reliability of the ADS. Based on the results of a factor analysis and internal consistency testing, the ADS was further reduced from 67 to 42 items.

DESCRIPTION OF THE ATTENTIONAL DEMANDS SURVEY

The final ADS (see Appendix at the end of this chapter) consists of 42 items encompassing demands within four theoretically derived domains:

TABLE 11.1 Studies Supporting the Reliability and Validity of the Attentional Demands Survey (ADS)

Study citation	Sample and characteristics	Reliability evidence	Validity evidence
Jansen, D. A., & Keller, M. L. (1998). Identifying the attentional demands perceived by elderly people. *Rehabilitation Nursing, 23*(1), 12–20.	*Sample size:* 30 *Sample characteristics:* Community-dwelling elderly 66 to 87 years of age (*M* = 76.6 years, *SD* = 5.3). 22 females (*M* = 77.1 years of age, *SD* = 6.0) and 8 males (*M* = 75.3 years of age, *SD* = 2.0). All were White and were born in the U.S. The first 15 participants resided in apartment buildings in a mid-sized midwestern city and the remaining 15 lived in houses in a small rural midwestern city. The urban participants were slightly older (*M* = 79.6 years of age, *SD* = 4.9) and better educated (*M* = 15.3 years, *SD* = 2.6) than the rural participants (*M* = 73.7 years of age, *SD* = 3.8; *M* = 12.8 years of education, *SD* = 2.7).	*Interrater:* Interview data were content analyzed for factors that serve as attentional demands. Specifically, the two researchers independently sorted each individual thought or theme expressed by a participant into the physical-environmental, informational, behavioral, and affective domains. Interrater reliability (percent agreement) when sorting by theoretical domains was 87.2%.	*A priori content validity:* Items for the ADS were developed from a content analysis of interview data: Elderly participants were interviewed regarding their perceptions of factors that serve as attentional demands within the physical-environmental, informational, behavioral, and affective domains. The open-ended questions and format of the interview were reviewed by knowledgeable researchers. The content analysis method outlined by McLaughlin and Marasculio (1990) was used to categorize the data into the four theorized domains. The themes within each domain were then worded into close-ended Likert-type scale items. *Posteriori content validity:* The items were reviewed by knowledgeable researchers for theoretical soundness and relevance, comprehensiveness, applicability to the elderly, and clarity and conciseness. Additionally, 4 elderly individuals participated in a pilot test of the instrument in order to provide feedback on its format and clarity. Based on the feedback from the researchers and the pilot test participants, the ADS was reduced from 92 items to 67.

TABLE 11.1 *(continued)*

Study citation	Sample and characteristics	Reliability evidence	Validity evidence
Jansen, D. A., & Keller, M. L. (1999). An instrument to measure the attentional demands of community-dwelling elders. *Journal of Nursing Measurement, 7*, 197–214.	*Sample size:* 197 *Sample characteristics:* Community-dwelling elderly 65 to 98 years of age ($M = 76.8$ years, $SD = 8.4$). 142 females ($M = 75.5$ years of age, $SD = 7.1$), 50 males ($M = 76.4$ years of age, $SD = 6.9$), and 5 participants did not specify gender. All were White and all except 5 were born in the U.S. At least 53% lived alone. Participants generally tended to be well educated with over 75% having completed high school or some college. All had normal mental status, as measured by the Short Portable Mental Status Questionnaire	*Test–retest.* The original 67-item version of the ADS was readministered following a 2-week interval to the first 26 participants who agreed to a retest. A Pearson r of .91 was obtained for the original 67-item version of the ADS. The Pearson r was .86 when only the final 42 retained items were considered. *Internal consistency:* The reliabilities (Cronbach's alpha) for the physical-environmental, informational, behavioral, and affective subscales were 0.87, 0.87, 0.87, and 0.90, respectively for the final 42-item version of the ADS Ranges for corrected item-scale correlations for each	*First factor analysis:* A factor analysis of the original 67-item version of the ADS was conducted using the Exploratory Factor Analysis Program (EFAP) by Joreskog and Sorbom (1978). A maximum likelihood method of extraction with Promax (oblique) rotations was employed to produce simple structure. A four-factor solution was the most interpretable, accounted for more variance, and produced simple structure. A scree test (Cattell, 1966) to evaluate the eigenvalues of the correlation matrix also indicated that the 4 factor solution was most appropriate. The factors corresponded to the theorized domains: physical-environmental, informational, behavioral, and affective. Deletion of Items: A total of 25 items were deleted from the 67-item ADS based on low factor loadings (less than .30), similar loadings on more than one factor, and high (greater than .70) inter-item correlations. *Second factor analysis:* A factor analysis of the remaining 42 items was repeated using the maximum likelihood method of extraction with a Promax rotation. The 4 factors emerged cleanly for 38 of the 42 items when the criterion for

TABLE 11.1 (*continued*)

Study citation	Sample and characteristics	Reliability evidence	Validity evidence
Jansen, D. A., & Keller, M. L. (1999) (*continued*)	(Pfeiffer, 1975). Participants were recruited from relatively rural (54%) and urban (46%) settings throughout a midwestern state.	domain were as follows: physical-environmental, .44–63; informational, .50–66; behavioral, .52–75; and affective, .45–74. Intercorrelations among the domain subscales ranged from .46 to .53.	loading was set at .40. The four remaining items loaded at .35 or greater and thus were retained. Ranges for the factor loadings were as follows: Physical-environmental, .38–66; informational, .38–86; behavioral, .35–80; and affective, .37–.81. The 4 factors accounted for 38% of the variance. Tucker's reliability coefficient was .92, an indication of the goodness of the fit of the data to the factor model.
Jansen, D. A., & Keller, M. L. (in press). Attentional demands and capacity to direct attention among elderly women. *Journal of Gerontological Nursing.*	*Sample size: 72* *Sample characteristics:* Community-dwelling elderly women drawn from a mid-sized midwestern city and its surrounding suburbs. 65–102 years of age ($M = 76.9$ years, $SD = 7.7$). 66 women were white and six were African American. All but two were born in the U.S. 78% were living alone; 75% resided in apartments and the remaining	*Internal consistency:* Cronbach's alpha estimates for the physical-environmental, informational, behavioral, and affective subscale domains were .80, .85, .80, and .83, respectively.	*Construct validity:* Hypothesis tested: Attentional demands will correlate negatively with performance on objective measures of CDA. Participants were administered the ADS along with a small battery of attention measures, including Digit Span Forward and Backward, the Symbol Digit Modalities Test, and the Trail Making Test parts A and B. Consistent with the hypothesis, a significant negative correlation ($r = -.31$, $p < .01$) was found between a total score for the ADS and a total attentional capacity score. Thus greater levels of attentional demands were associated with more difficulty directing attention. Correlations between each of the subscales and the total attentional capacity score were $r = -.18$ for physical environmental, $r = -.25$ ($p < .05$) for informational, $r = -.20$ for behavioral, and $r = -.37$ ($p \leq .01$) for the affective domain.

TABLE 11.1 *(continued)*

Study citation	Sample and characteristics	Reliability evidence	Validity evidence
	25% lived in houses. The women averaged 14.2 years ($SD = 2.8$) of formal education. Participants tended to be healthy and described a relatively low level of attentional demands (ADS total score $M = 54.3$, $SD = 26.1$, Range = 18–124). Subscale ADS means were as follows: physical-environmental, $M = 20.1$ ($SD = 9.9$); informational, $M = 11.8$ ($SD = 8.1$); behavioral, $M = 6.5$ ($SD = 5.5$); and affective, $M = 15.9$ ($SD = 8.5$).		

physical-environmental (items 1–14), informational (items 15–25), behavioral (items 26–31), and affective (items 32–42). The participant rates each item using a 5–point Likert-type scale ranging from 0 = *not at all* to 4 = *a lot* in terms of how much the situation described "takes effort or makes life difficult." Both phrases were used because any situation perceived as "taking effort" or "making life difficult" requires CDA and thus creates attentional demands.

SCORING OF THE ATTENTIONAL DEMANDS SURVEY

Because the four domains are different but related dimensions of the concept of attentional demands, item scores within each domain are summed to create subscale totals. Higher scores reflect exposure to greater intensities of attentional demands and thus increased risk for developing DAF. Maximum attainable scores for each of the subscales are 56, 44, 24, and 44, respectively, for the physical-environmental, informational, behavioral, and affective domains. Summing the subscales may produce a total possible score of 168. To reduce potential demands caused by decreased visual acuity, it is recommended that at least a size 14 font be used when administering the instrument to the elderly.

CONCLUSIONS AND RECOMMENDATIONS

Presently, the ADS meets Norbeck's (1985) criteria for a usable instrument. That is, minimally, an instrument should possess content validity, test-retest reliability, and internal consistency, along with at least one type of construct or criterion-related validity. Interviews with community-dwelling elderly participants, a content analysis, and reviews of the items by experts provided support for the content validity of the ADS (Jansen & Keller, 1998). In a second study (Jansen & Keller, 1999) aimed at determining the psychometric properties of the ADS, test–retest and internal consistency reliabilities reached acceptable levels and a factor analysis provided some evidence for construct validity. In a third study (Jansen & Keller, in press), a significant negative correlation was found between attentional demands and CDA. This finding of higher levels of attentional demands being associated with greater difficulty with attention measures is consistent with a theoretically derived hypothesis and thus provides further evidence for construct validity.

A number of limitations in the present studies need to be considered when using the ADS and in designing future studies. To date, the ADS has been tested with predominantly white, community-dwelling, elderly Midwestern women and a few men. More research is needed with elderly men and older people from more culturally diverse populations. Testing the ADS with people experiencing higher levels of attentional demands also is necessary, as item means tended to be relatively low. Higher levels of demands may not have been reported because all the participants in the three described studies were self-selected, and thus it is likely that those people with better attentional functioning and lower, more manageable levels of attentional demands chose to be in the research samples. Additionally, another limitation concerns the occurrence of missing data for the ADS in the study (Jansen & Keller, 1999) aimed at determining the psychometric properties of the instrument. This was handled via mean substitution for individual domains. Finally, due to the newness of the ADS and its limited testing and use to date, replication involving confirmatory factor analysis is desirable for further verification of the factor structure (Gorsuch, 1983) and other psychometric properties.

REFERENCES

Bjorklund, D. F., & Harnishfeger, K. K. (1995). The evolution of inhibition mechanisms and their role in human cognition and behavior. In F. N. Dempster & C. J. Brainerd (Eds.), *Interference and inhibition in cognition* (pp. 141–173). San Diego, CA: Academic Press.

Brown, L. A., Shumway-Cook, A., & Woollacott, M. H. (1999). Attentional demands and postural recovery: The effects of aging. *Journal of Gerontology: Medical Sciences, 54A,* M165–M171.

Cattell, R. B. (1966). The scree test for the number of factors. *Multivariate Behavioral Research, 1,* 245–276.

Cimprich, B. (1992a). Attentional fatigue following breast cancer surgery. *Research in Nursing & Health, 15,* 199–207.

Cimprich, B. (1992b). A theoretical perspective on attention and patient education. *Advances in Nursing Science, 14*(3), 39–51.

Cimprich, B. (1993a). [Evaluating usefulness of tests of attentional capacity in healthy adults]. Unpublished raw data.

Cimprich, B. (1993b). Development of an intervention to restore attention in cancer patients. *Cancer Nursing, 16,* 83–92.

Cimprich, B. (1995). Symptom management: Loss of concentration. *Seminars in Oncology Nursing, 11,* 279–288.

Cimprich, B. (1998). Age and extent of surgery affect attention in women treated for breast cancer. *Research in Nursing & Health, 21,* 229–238.

Gorsuch, R. L. (1983). *Factor analysis* (2nd ed.). Hillsdale, NJ: Erlbaum.

Jansen, D. A. (1997). *Attentional demands and restorative activities: Do they influence directed attention among the elderly?* Unpublished doctoral dissertation, University of Wisconsin, Madison.

Jansen, D. A., & Cimprich. B. (1994). Attentional impairment in persons with multiple sclerosis. *Journal of Neuroscience Nursing, 26,* 95–102.

Jansen, D. A., & Keller, M. L. (1998). Identifying the attentional demands perceived by elderly people. *Rehabilitation Nursing, 23*(1), 12–20.

Jansen, D. A., & Keller, M. L. (1999). An instrument to measure the attentional demands of community-dwelling elders. *Journal of Nursing Measurement, 7*, 197–214.

Jansen, D. A., & Keller, M. L. (in press). Attentional demands and capacity to direct attention among elderly women. *Journal of Gerontological Nursing.*

Joreskog, K. G., & Sorbom, D. (1978). *EFAP Exploratory factor analysis program: User's guide.* Chicago, IL: International Educational Services.

Kaplan, R., & Kaplan, S. (1989). *The experience of nature: A psychological perspective.* New York: Cambridge University Press.

Kaplan, S. (1995). The restorative benefits of nature: Toward an integrative framework. *Journal of Environmental Psychology, 15*, 169–182.

Kaplan, S., & Kaplan, R. (1983). *Cognition and environment.* New York: Praeger.

Lezak, M. D. (1995). *Neuropsychological assessment* (3rd ed.). New York: Oxford University Press.

McDowd, J. M., & Shaw, R. J. (2000). Attention and aging: A functional perspective. In F. I. M. Craik & T. A. Salthouse (Eds.), *The handbook of aging and cognition* (2nd ed., pp. 221–292). Mahwah, NJ: Erlbaum.

McKnight, A. J., & McKnight, A. S. (1999). Multivariate analysis of age-related driver ability and performance deficits. *Accident Analysis and Prevention, 31*, 445–454.

McLaughlin, F. E., & Marascuilo, L. A. (1990). *Advanced nursing and health care research.* Philadelphia: Saunders.

Mesulam, M. M. (1985). Attention, confusional states, and neglect. In M. M. Mesulam (Ed.), *Principles of behavioral neurology* (pp. 125–167). Philadelphia: Davis.

Norbeck, J. S. (1985). What constitutes a publishable report of instrument development? *Nursing Research, 34*, 380–382.

Parasuraman, R., & Greenwood, P. M. (1998). Selective attention in aging and dementia. In R. Parasuraman (Ed.), *The attentive brain* (pp. 461–487). Cambridge, MA: MIT Press.

Pfeiffer, E. (1975). A short portable mental status questionnaire for the assessment of organic brain deficit in elderly patients. *Journal of the American Geriatrics Society, 23*, 433–441.

Raz, N. (2000). Aging of the brain and its impact on cognitive performance: Integration of structural and functional findings. In F. I. M. Craik & T. A. Salthouse (Eds.), *The handbook of aging and cognition* (2nd ed., pp. 1–90). Mahwah, NJ: Erlbaum.

Reuter-Lorenz, P. A. (2000). Cognitive neuropsychology of the brain. In D. Park & N. Schwarz (Eds.), *Cognitive aging* (pp. 93–114). Philadelphia: Psychology Press.

Tun, P. A. (1998). Fast noisy speech: Age differences in processing rapid speech with background noise. *Psychology and Aging, 13,* 424–434.

van Zomeren, A. H., & Brouwer, W. H. (1994). *Clinical neuropsychology of attention.* New York: Oxford University Press.

von Hippel, W., Silver, L. A., & Lynch, M. E. (2000). Stereotyping against your will: The role of inhibitory ability in stereotyping and prejudice among the elderly. *Personality and Social Psychology Bulletin, 26,* 523–532.

Wegner, D. M. (1989). *White bears and other unwanted thoughts.* New York: Viking.

Wegner, D. M., & Erber, R. (1992). The hyperaccessibility of suppressed thoughts. *Journal of Personality and Social Psychology, 63,* 903–912.

APPENDIX: ATTENTIONAL DEMANDS SURVEY

This questionnaire lists things that many people face in their daily lives. Some of the items on the list may not affect you. However, people find that a number of these things use physical or mental energy because they take effort or make their lives difficult.

Each item is followed by a scale that goes from "Not at all" (0) to "A lot" (4).

For each item on the questionnaire, you will be asked to circle the number that shows how much each of these things takes effort or makes day-to-day life difficult.

Here is an example: If uncomfortable or harsh weather conditions make life a lot harder, circle "4". Your answer would look like this:

Takes Effort or Makes Life Difficult

Not at all		Somewhat		A lot
0	1	2	3	4

1.   Uncomfortable or harsh weather conditions
        0   1   2   3   ④

The following items are things in the physical environment that may affect your day-to-day life. Please circle only one number for each item:

Takes Effort or Makes Life Difficult

Not at all		Somewhat		A lot
0	1	2	3	4

1. Uncomfortable or harsh weather conditions
        0   1   2   3   4
2. Noise distractions
        0   1   2   3   4
3. Bright sunlight and glare
        0   1   2   3   4
4. Not enough light
        0   1   2   3   4
5. Outside obstacles such as construction sites and hills
        0   1   2   3   4
6. Not enough living space
        0   1   2   3   4
7. Building construction such as stairs and long distances
        0   1   2   3   4

Takes Effort or Makes Life Difficult

Not at all   **Somewhat**   **A lot**

0   **1**   **2**   **3**   **4**

8. The design of furniture and appliances
   0   1   2   3   4

9. Buildings that are hard to find your way around in
   0   1   2   3   4

10. Things having to do with driving
    0   1   2   3   4

11. Things having to do with being a passenger in a car
    0   1   2   3   4
12. Too much going on at once
    0   1   2   3   4

13. Dealing with new, unfamiliar, or changed situations
    0   1   2   3   4
14. Having to move
    0   1   2   3   4

The following items are things that require you to deal with information or may affect your ability to deal with information in day-to-day living. Please circle only one number for each item:

15. Takes longer to understand what you read
    0   1   2   3   4
16. Distracted by own thoughts
    0   1   2   3   4
17. Conflicting or unclear information, such as with taxes, bank statements, doctor appointments
    0   1   2   3   4
18. Trouble following what people say to you
    0   1   2   3   4
19. Trouble with memory and forgetfulness
    0   1   2   3   4
20. Trouble hearing
    0   1   2   3   4
21. Trouble seeing
    0   1   2   3   4
22. Reading or responding to the mail
    0   1   2   3   4

Takes Effort or Makes Life Difficult

Not at all   **Somewhat**   **A lot**

0   **1**   **2**   **3**   **4**

23. Going to the doctor or clinic or special appointments
    0   1   2   3   4
24. Sorting and organizing belongings
    0   1   2   3   4
25. Managing medications
    0   1   2   3   4

The following items are things that make it difficult for you to do what you want or need to do. Please circle only one number for each item:

26. Being forced to wait, such as for rides or at appointments
    0   1   2   3   4
27. Financial restrictions
    0   1   2   3   4
28. Lack or loss of privacy
    0   1   2   3   4
29. Giving up independence or control over life
    0   1   2   3   4
30. Not free to express your thoughts or feelings
    0   1   2   3   4
31. Other people do not listen or understand you
    0   1   2   3   4

The following items involve feelings and concerns that affect day-to-day life for some people. Please circle only one number for each item:

Takes Effort or Makes Life Difficult

Not at all   **Somewhat**   **A lot**

0   **1**   **2**   **3**   **4**

32. Pain and discomfort
    0   1   2   3   4
33. Health problems
    0   1   2   3   4
34. Being alone or isolated
    0   1   2   3   4
35. Worries about the future of society
    0   1   2   3   4

Takes Effort or Makes Life Difficult

Not at all		Somewhat		A lot
0	1	2	3	4

36. Fear of falling
        0   1   2   3   4
37. Worries about your own health
        0   1   2   3   4
38. Feeling sad about your present life situation
        0   1   2   3   4
39. Missing activities or work that you used to do
        0   1   2   3   4
40. Missing the past
        0   1   2   3   4
41. Missing family or friends who have died or live far away
        0   1   2   3   4
42. Worries about health and future of friends or family
        0   1   2   3   4

PART II

Client's Perceptions of Care

12

Measuring Distress During Painful Medical Procedures: The Distress Checklist

Nancy Wells

This chapter discusses the Distress Checklist, an observational measure of distress during painful medical procedures in adults.

PURPOSE

The Distress Checklist was developed to measure behavioral indicators of distress during a painful and anxiety-producing procedure (Wells, 1990). An observational measure, this instrument assesses the four dimensions of negative emotion proposed by Davitz (1969) hyperactivation, tension, moving against, and inadequacy, and the four categories of emotional behavior: facial expression, posture, vocalization, and verbalization (Groen, 1975; Klinger, 1982).

CONCEPTUAL BASIS OF THE DISTRESS CHECKLIST

Johnson (Johnson, 1972, 1973; Johnson & Rice, 1974) built her definition of distress on Beecher's model of pain, emphasizing the unpleasant quality of the emotional state. Leventhal and Johnson (1983) explicitly delineated the behaviors associated with emotional response (including distress) as subjective report of emotional state, expressive reaction, postural changes indicative of tension, and psychophysiologic reactions. Behavioral measures of emotion include one or more of the following categories: facial expression, posture, vocalization, and verbalization (Groen, 1975; Klinger, 1982).

The conceptual basis of the Distress Checklist was approached within a framework of emotional meaning, as developed by Davitz (1969). Four dimensions of emotion were defined, with a positive pole and two negative poles describing distinct negative emotional patterns. The four dimensions include activation (level of energy and arousal), unpleasantness, relatedness to the environment (approach-avoidance), and competence (a sense of how well one is adapting to the environment) (Davitz). The dimensions of activation and unpleasantness reflect internal, feeling states, whereas relatedness and competence reflect interaction with the environment. The essential characteristics of distress include the perception of threat, giving rise to a transitory negative emotional state that is described as unpleasant. This emotional state may be modified by cognition (i.e., incompetence, inadequacy, competence). The primary function of distress is to communicate the feeling of unpleasantness to self and others (Tomkins, 1984).

PROCEDURES FOR DEVELOPMENT

The behaviors selected were drawn from previous research. Twelve items were derived from the literature and direct observation of women during a painful surgical procedure—abortion. For example, behaviors reflecting tension included tension around eyes and mouth and expression reflecting pain and anxiety. Vocalization was limited to grunts, groans, and sighs, whereas verbalization was spoken words. Following content validity determination, two items were added (crying and lack of eye contact). For clarity, the behaviors were grouped according to the four parameters of emotional measurement, that is, facial expression, posture, vocalization, and verbalization. The number of items on the final version of the checklist was reduced to seven based on the results of field testing.

DESCRIPTION

The Distress Checklist is a compilation of seven behaviors that can be observed when a person is in distress. The observer, who rates the behaviors, is provided operational definitions for each of the seven behaviors to ensure consistency of ratings by ensuring a common interpretation of each item on the checklist. Spaces are provided beside each listed behavior for the rater to note whether the behavior was observed or was absent. The Distress Checklist will be found in the Appendix at the end of this chapter.

ADMINISTRATION AND SCORING

The Distress Checklist requires between five to seven minutes to complete, depending upon the length of the procedure. The rater observes the patient during the medical procedure and notes whether each of the seven behaviors on the checklist is observed within that time frame. The behaviors that are noted as present by the observer are summed for a total behavioral distress score. Although scoring of the actual behavior is criterion-based, the sum of behaviors exhibited places the subject on a continuum of scores that range from 0 to 7. Thus, higher scores reflect greater behavioral distress.

RELIABILITY AND VALIDITY EVIDENCE

Reliability and validity of the Distress Checklist were determined on a sample of 36 women undergoing first trimester abortion. Following content validation by eight health care professionals, a correlational design was used to determine concurrent and discriminant validity. Concurrent validity was examined by the correlation among distress measures from three response modes: behavioral, subjective, and physiological. To discriminate behavioral distress from related concepts of pain and anxiety, the state anxiety scale of the State-Trait Anxiety Inventory (STAI) (Spielberger, Gorush, Lushene, Vagg, & Jacobs, 1983) and the McGill Pain Questionnaire (MPQ) (Melzack, 1975) were administered. Construct validity also was tested using the contrasted-groups approach. It was hypothesized that subjects undergoing abortion with local anesthesia would experience more distress as measured on the Distress Checklist than subjects undergoing abortion with IV sedation.

PROCEDURE

Following consent to participate, the subject completed the 20–item state anxiety scale from the STAI (Spielberger et al., 1983). A baseline pulse was then obtained. These measures were collected 30 to 90 minutes prior to the abortion procedure. During the procedure, the subject's behaviors were rated by an observer using the Distress Checklist. On completion of the procedure, the subject completed the sensory and distress visual analogue scales (VASs), and an independent observer who was unaware of the content of the Distress Checklist completed a distress VAS. Once the subject was admitted to the recovery room, the MPQ was administered using an interview format (Melzack, 1975, 1983).

Sample

A convenience sample of 39 women were recruited from a private abortion clinic. Of these subjects, data from five women undergoing abortion with local anesthesia were used to determine interrater reliability. Of the remaining 34 subjects, 31 women with complete data comprised the sample for reliability and validity testing. The mean age of the sample was 26 years (SD = 6.2). Forty-five percent of the women had some college education.

McGill Pain Questionnaire

The MPQ was used to measure intensity of pain, using the Pain Rating Index (PRI) total score and the Present Pain Intensity (PPI). The PRI also may be divided into three subscales tapping sensory, affective, and evaluative dimensions of pain. Internal consistency of the PRI total was adequate in this sample (alpha = 0.84). Because of the questionable validity of the MPQ subscales (Turk, Rudy, & Salovey, 1985), the PRI total score was used as a measure of pain intensity.

State Anxiety

State anxiety was measured with the A-state of the State-Trait Anxiety Inventory (STAI), Form Y-1 (Spielberger et al., 1983). Mean internal consistency of the A-state across different age and gender groups is 0.93; similar internal consistency was found in the present study (alpha = 0.91). Validity of the A-state was supported by the predicted decline from pre- to postsurgery (e.g., Auerbach, 1973; Spielberger, Auerbach, Wadsworth, Dunn, & Taulbee, 1973).

Self-Report of Pain Sensation and Distress

Pain sensation and distress were obtained on two visual analogue scales. The value in millimeters was obtained by measuring from the left, zero, position to the subject's mark. The mean pain sensation was 53.48 (SD = 28.0), with a range from 0 to 100. Distress was slightly lower, with a mean of 45.74 (SD = 27.58) and a range from 1 to 98. The variability of both subjective measures is large.

Observer-Rated Distress

An independent observer, who was unaware of the specific items on the Distress Checklist, rated the subject's distress on a VAS. Mean observer-rated distress was 33.40 (SD = 25.11), with a range from 1 to 90. Again, variability of this measure is large.

Interrater Reliability

Five subjects were observed by the investigator and a trained research assistant. Interrater agreement on behaviors exhibited by women undergoing abortion with local anesthesia reached 100% on the Distress Checklist for the final two subjects. Mean interrater correlation was $r = .90$, with only two items correlated less than 1.00. Thus, interrater reliability was supported.

Internal Consistency

Internal consistency was determined by interitem correlations and the KR-20. Several items had no variance over the 31 subjects and were deleted from the analysis. These items included restlessness, verbal anxiety, and lack of coping. The KR-20 for the remaining 11 items was .60. Lack of eye contact was negatively correlated with most of the other distress behaviors.

Three additional items had low item-to-total correlations (knees pulled together, crying, and requests for emotional support); these items were deleted from the analysis. The remaining seven items were adequately intercorrelated, providing a KR-20 of .71. Item-to-total correlations ranged from .26 to .60.

Concurrent Validity

Concurrent validity is supported by the degree of association among the distress measures. Behavioral distress was significantly and positively correlated with self-reported distress ($r = .35$, $p = .05$) and observer-rated distress ($r = .74$, $p = .01$) using Pearson correlation procedures. The PPI, which Melzack (1975) suggests is influenced by the emotional dimension of pain, was also significantly correlated with behavioral distress ($p = .40$).

The magnitude of correlations between self-report and observational measures of distress is moderate, explaining 12% to 16% of variance. The observer-rated correlation is stronger, and accounts for 55% of the variance in the Distress Checklist score. This suggests a communicative function of behavioral distress as measured by the Distress Checklist. Heart rate at Time 2, controlling for Time 1, was not related to any of the observed or subjective distress measures.

Construct Validity

Measures of state anxiety and pain intensity were used to determine whether behavioral distress is adequately differentiated from these concepts. Behavioral distress was significantly and positively correlated with self-report of pain sensation on the VAS (p = .51, p = .01). This correlation was stronger than the correlation between behavioral and self-reported distress. The correlation between self-reported sensation and distress was r = .66, suggesting a degree of overlap in these two measures. This may be related to the method of measurement or an inadequate explanation of the difference between these concepts to the subject. Behavioral distress was not related to state anxiety or pain intensity measured by the PRI total. These findings support the notion that behavioral distress is distinct from state anxiety and pain intensity. The intercorrelation between VAS measures of sensation and distress requires further investigation.

Construct Validity Assessment through Contrasted-Groups Approach

The final method of determining construct validity was the contrasted-groups approach. It was hypothesized that women undergoing abortion with local anesthesia would exhibit more behavioral distress than women undergoing abortion with IV sedation. As hypothesized, women undergoing abortion with local anesthesia scored significantly higher on the Distress Checklist than women receiving IV sedation [t (29) = 2.99, p = .006]. Thus, construct validity of the Distress Checklist was supported by the mean differences found by type of anesthesia.

SUMMARY AND CONCLUSIONS

The Distress Checklist was tested on a sample of 31 women undergoing first trimester uncomplicated abortion. The revised, seven-item Distress Checklist demonstrated adequate internal consistency for a newly developed instrument. Several aspects of construct validity were supported; however, the deletion of half of the original items suggests inconsistency between conceptual and empirical definitions.

The revisions in the Distress Checklist significantly alter the content of the instrument. This suggests that conceptual development is inconsistent with the obtained empirical data based on observation. The majority of items retained (five of the seven) assessed the tension class of hedonic tone, thus sampling only the hyperactive (i.e., anxiety-related) dimension of emotion, which is more amenable to observation. However, the lack of correlation between behavioral distress and preabortion state anxiety suggests these are two distinct phenomena; the distinction may be related to response mode (i.e., behavioral observation and self-report) or the presence of pain. Retrospective reports of anxiety during the procedure might have resulted in a correlation with observed distress, however. Thus, the

Distress Checklist may assess the hyperactive dimension of emotional response directly related to pain, whereas state anxiety a measured in this study is more generally related to the entire situation. Despite low association between these two measures, state anxiety was a predictor of behavioral distress. Consistent with the literature on acute pain, anxiety was a major intervening variable in this sample.

The conceptual-empirical inconsistencies of the Distress Checklist suggest that it measures a specific type of distress: pain-related distress, which, in this sample, is distinct from but influenced by state anxiety. The strong correlation between observer ratings and behavioral distress indicates the communicative function of this concept.

The items retained on the Distress Checklist reflect increased muscle tension and vocalization related to pain. The items not retained reflect, in general, higher levels of distress. One item, lack of eye contact, was negatively correlated with the total scale score. Lack of eye contact could be reflective of withdrawal or moving away and may be conceived of as a means of coping with pain. Restlessness, verbal anxiety, and lack of coping had no variance in this sample. Crying, the final item deleted, was a poor discriminator of distress in this setting. It is possible that this was not considered a socially acceptable response by subjects and therefore was not exhibited.

Construct validity was supported by the significantly higher behavioral distress scores; by the distinction found between distress, pain intensity, and state anxiety; and by the significantly higher behavioral distress scores of women undergoing abortion with local anesthesia as compared to IV sedation. In conclusion, the Distress Checklist has demonstrated adequate preliminary reliability and validity. This instrument shows promise as a valid observational measure of distress during medical procedures such as abortion. Further testing in different populations may produce a useful observational outcome measure in nursing research.

ACKNOWLEDGMENT

This study was supported by Public Health Service National Research Service Award No. F31–NU05928. The assistance of Mary Derby, BS, Geraldine Padilla, PhD, and the staff of Preterm Reproductive Health Clinic is acknowledged.

REFERENCES

Auerbach, S. M. (1973). Trait-state anxiety and adjustment to surgery. *Journal of Consulting and Clinical Psychology, 40,* 264–271.
Davitz, J. R. (1969). *The language of emotion.* New York: Academic.

Groen, J. J. (1975). The measurement of emotion and arousal in the clinical psychological laboratory and in medical practice. In L. Levi (Ed.), *Emotions: Their parameters and measurement* (pp. 727–746). New York: Raven Press.

Johnson, J. E. (1972). Effects of structuring patients' expectations on their reactions to threatening events. *Nursing Research, 21,* 499–504.

Johnson, J. E. (1973). Effects of accurate expectations about sensory and distress components of pain. *Journal of Personality and Social Psychology, 27,* 261–275.

Johnson, J. E., & Rice, V. H. (1974). Sensory and distress components of pain: Implications for the study of clinical pain. *Nursing Research, 23,* 203–209.

Klinger, E. (1982). On the self-management of mood, affect, and attention. In P. Karoly & F. H. Kanfer (Eds.), *Self-management and behavior change: From theory to practice* (pp. 129–164). New York: Pergamon.

Leventhal, H., & Johnson, J. E. (1983). Laboratory and field experimentation: Development of a theory of self-regulation. In P. Wooldridge, M. Schmitt, J. Skipper, & R. Leonard (Eds.), *Behavioral science and nursing theory* (pp. 189–262). St. Louis: Mosby.

Melzack, R. (1975). The McGill Pain Questionnaire: Major properties and scoring methods. *Pain, 1,* 277–299.

Melzack, R. (1983). The McGill Pain Questionnaire. In R. Melzack (Ed.), *Pain measurement and assessment* (pp. 41–48). New York: Raven Press.

Spielberger, C. D., Auerbach, S. M., Wadsworth, A. P., Dunn, T. M., & Taulbee, E. S. (1973). Emotional reactions to surgery. *Journal of Consulting and Clinical Psychology, 40,* 33–38.

Spielberger, C. D., Gorush, R. L., Lushene, R. E., Vagg, P. R., & Jacobs, G. A. (1983). STAI *Manual for the State-Trait Anxiety Inventory (Form Y).* Palo Alto, CA: Consulting Psychologists Press.

Tomkins, S. S. (1984). Affect theory. In K. R. Scherer & P. Ekman (Eds.), *Approaches to emotion* (pp. 163–195). Hillsdale, NJ: Erlbaum.

Turk, D. C., Rudy, T. E., & Salovey, P. (1985). The McGill Pain Questionnaire: Confirming the factor structure and examining appropriate uses. *Pain, 21,* 385–397.

Wells, N. (1990). Behavioral measurement of distress during painful medical procedures. In O.L. Strickland, & C. F. Waltz (Eds.), *Measurement of nursing outcomes (Vol. 4): Measuring client self-care and coping skills* (pp. 250–266). New York: Springer Publishing Co.

APPENDIX: DISTRESS CHECKLIST

Start _____   Finish _____
Pulse _____

Directions: Check whether each of the behaviors below were observed during the health care procedure by checking "present." If the behavior was *not* observed, leave the item blank.

		Present
1.	Tension around eyes	_____
2.	Tension around mouth	_____
3.	Flinch (sudden jerk)	_____
4.	Fists clenched/clutching	_____
5.	Audible expiration (sigh, grunt)	_____
6.	Pain expression (oh, ouch, groan)	_____
7.	Requests termination	_____
	Total	_____

COMMENTS:

Operational Definitions

1. Tension around eyes: eyes squeezed closed, flutter or wrinkle in eyelids
2. Tension around mouth: tightened lips, chin puckered or jaw clenched
3. Flinch: brief, sudden jerk of torso
4. Fists clenched/clutching: fists tight, may have white knuckles, or clutching gown, table, or other's hand
5. Audible expiration: audible expiration of sound; sigh, grunt
6. Pain expression: vocal expression of pain: oh, ouch, groan
7. Requests termination: states "stop," "I can't take this"

Administration and Scoring

Time of observation: Observation begins as the procedure begins. Time is recorded, and the subject is observed for the occurrence of the 7 behaviors until the procedure ends. Finish time is recorded. Each behavior can only be scored once.

Scoring: Each behavior is equally weighted, and scored as absent (0) or present (1). The total distress score is the sum, ranging from 0 (no distress) to 7 (extreme distress).

13

The Child Medical Fears Scale

Marion E. Broome and Teri Mobley

This chapter discusses the Child Medical Fear Scale, a measure of children's concerns about health care experiences.

PURPOSE

Children's responses to health care experiences have been a concern of health care providers and researchers for several decades (Hart & Bossert, 1994; Thompson, 1985; Vernon, Foley, Sipowitz, & Schulman, 1965). Much nursing research has been directed toward developing a better understanding of children's responses to stressful medical experiences in order to develop effective interventions to ameliorate stress (Broome & Huth, 2000; Melnyk, 1994). Although many children respond to stressful medical events with distress, others do not. Intrinsic characteristics, such as fear of medical experiences, have been documented to be one variable that influences their response to a variety of experiences in health care (Abu-Saad, Pool, & Tulkens, 1994; Beyer & Knott, 1998; Bournaki, 1997; Broome, Bates, Lillis, & McGahee, 1992; Wilson & Yorker, 1997). The purpose of this chapter is to describe the initial development and testing of the Child Medical Fear Scale (CMFS), as well as the empirical evidence supporting the reliability and validity of the scale.

CONCEPTUAL BASIS FOR THE CMFS

There are several theoretical perspectives that provide some understanding of the epigenesis of childhood fears (Nicastro & Whetsell, 1999). These include traditional psychoanalytic theory, social learning theory, Piaget's theory of cognitive development and differentiation theory (Freud, 1856; Lerner, 1997; Piaget, 1896/1967; Witkin, 1974). Although initially it appears that these theoretical perspectives posit different explanations for why children become fearful of selected experiences, there are several concepts common to these various theories that provided a basis for the development of a tool that measures children's fears of medical experiences.

Fear is a normal developmental characteristic. It has been defined as a specific biological and psychological response to a very real or imagined threat (Nicastro & Whetsell, 1999). Medical fears are defined as "any experience that involves medical personnel or procedures involved in the process of evaluating or modifying health status in traditional health care settings" (Steward & Steward, 1981, p. 70).

Fear as an innate response requires a certain level of maturation and differentiation in the human child. When the child perceives him/herself differentiated from the environment, is cognitively mature enough to perceive a threat to self, interacts with the environment during a stressful experience and perceives a threat to self (initial response), the child learns to fear that specific threatening event or person. This learning results in new emotional and biological responses evidenced by the child that are designed to evade the feared experience in the future. When the experience cannot be evaded, this fear will become evident in greater levels of evasion, behavioral distress, and anxiety.

Health care experiences, in general, are threatening to preschool and school age children. Health care experiences often involve separating children from family, friends, and familiar environments. Invasion of the child's privacy and threats to body integrity are not uncommon (Broome & Huth, 2000). All of these experiences are threatening to children and will, depending on the child, produce some level of fear of medical experiences.

PROCEDURES FOR DEVELOPMENT

Two studies were conducted during the initial development of the CMFS (Broome, Hellier, Wilson, Dale & Glanville, 1988). The first involved interviewing 146 well, school-age children who responded to questions asking how it felt to be sick and to interact with doctors and nurses, what they liked and disliked about being sick, and how they felt when they had to go to the hospital. Each interview took 15 minutes and the taped interviews were analyzed. Four themes were initially identified from the interviews and twenty-nine items were developed that addressed all four themes. The themes were fears related to interactions with health care professionals (n = 9 items), their own bodies (n = 4), medical procedures (n = 9) and the health care environment (n = 7).

In the second study, the CMFS was administered to 84 additional well, school-age children in order to test the psychometric properties of the instrument and examine the feasibility of the administration procedures (Table 13.1). The CMFS demonstrated adequate reliability and validity.

An item analysis revealed high correlations (> .70) among the four sub-scales. This indicated that in this sample the subscales were not independent and were likely measuring overlapping concepts. Therefore, it was suggested that further testing be done before these subscales were used in future studies. In subsequent testing of the CMFS with small samples of acutely ill children and a study of children with cancer (Broome et al., 1992), redundant items with little variability or those that had a high correlation with another item were eliminated, thus reducing the number of items on the CMFS to 17.

DESCRIPTION

The Child Medical Fear Scale (Appendix) consists of 17 items. The child is asked to rate, on a three-point scale, how afraid he/she is of selected experiences associated with health care. The response format recommended for school-age children is 0 = *not at all afraid,* 1 = *a little afraid,* 2 = *a lot afraid.* There is also a CMFS-parent version for researchers to administer to parents to elicit their perception about how afraid their child is of medical experiences (Broome, 1999). The CMFS-child version has been translated into three languages: Dutch (Abu-Saad et al., 1994), Thai (Chaiyawat, 2000), and Chinese. The Thai and Chinese versions are available in The CMFS Manual (Broome, 1999).

ADMINISTRATION AND SCORING

The CMFS can be given to the child over 6 years of age to complete, but more often researchers have asked the child to answer the questions during an interview. The child is asked to indicate how much fear he/she has of selected medical experiences. Each item can be scored as 0 = *none,* 1 = *a little* or 2 = *a lot.* There are no reversed scored items. The range of the possible scores on the 17–item CMFS is 0 to 34. Low scores mean less fear, while high scores mean greater fear. In a recent study by Beyer and Knott (1998), the CMFS was used with preschool children and the response format was changed such that they could indicate which of various sized circles reflected how afraid they were. Beyer and Knott (1998) report additional psychometric testing on the version used with younger children.

RELIABILITY AND VALIDITY EVIDENCE

The CMFS has been used to study children's fears of medical experiences in six published studies from 1992–1998, as well as a variety of unpub-

TABLE 13.1 Published Studies Using Child Medical Fear Scale

Study citation	CMFS version	Sample and characteristics	Reliability evidence	Validity evidence
Broome, M.E., Hellier, A., Wilson, T., Dale, S., & Glanville, C. (1988). Measuring children's fear of medical experiences. In C. F. Waltz & O. L. Strickland (Eds.), *Measurement of nursing outcomes* (Vol 1, pp. 201–214). New York: Springer.	29-item original Child Medical Fear Scale was used to identify how individual children vary in their degree of fearfulness of medical experiences.	*Sample size:* 146 children. *Sample Characteristics:* 6 to 11 years of age. 71% Caucasian; 48% males.	*Internal consistency:* Cronbach's alpha = .93 for total test.	*Content validity:* 78% *Criterion validity:* Significant correlation between the Medical Fear Subscale and CMFS, $r = .71$ ($p < .001$) *Discriminant validity:* No significant relationship between age of a child and CMFS score, $r = .04$ ($p > .05$).
Broome, M. E., Bates, T. A., Lillis, P. P., & McGahee, T. W. (1992). Children's medical fears, coping behaviors, and pain perceptions during a lumbar puncture. *Oncology Nursing Forum, 17,* 361–367.	29-item CMFS was used to identify the relationship among medical fear, coping behaviors, and acute pain perceptions in children with cancer.	*Sample size:* 17 children. *Sample characteristics:* 3 and 15 years of age. 14 boys and 3 girls.	*Internal consistency:* Cronbach's alpha = .93 for the total test	*Criterion validity:* Moderately positive relationship between medical fear and pain ratings, $r = .54$ ($p = .01$) *Discriminant validity:* No significant differences were found between medical fear levels children exhibit and active or passive coping behaviors.
Abu-Saad, J. J., Pool, M., & Tulkens, B. (1994). Further validity testing of	The 17-item CMFS was translated for use by an official	*First study:* *Sample size:* 26 children, 11 boys	*Internal consistency:* Cronbach's alpha = .93 for total scale	*Content validity:* Reviewed by 2 experts who determined appropriate

TABLE 13.1 (*continued*)

Study citation	CMFS version	Sample and characteristics	Reliability evidence	Validity evidence
the Abu-Saad Paediatric Pain Assessment Tool. *Journal of Advanced Nursing, 19,* 1063–1071.	Dutch translator in 3 steps (English to Dutch, Dutch to English, and English to Dutch).	and 15 girls. *Second study*: *Sample size*: 79 children, 47 boys and 32 girls. *Sample characteristics*: 5 to 15 years; hospitalized for medical or surgical procedures, had analgesic medication prescribed.	Cronbach's alpha for Environmental = .78 Procedural = .66	ness for Dutch children. *Criterion validity*: Scores on pain tool and CMFS correlated. Pain and environmental fear correlated = .18 ($p < .05$); procedural = .23 ($p < .01$) *Discriminant validity*: No differences in fear scores were found in relation to previous hospital experience and gender. *Factor analysis*: Environmental fears = 21.8% of variance; Procedural fears, 8.7% of variance in pain scores.
Hart, D., & Bossert, E. (1994). Self-reported fears of hospitalized school-age children. *Journal of Pediatric Nursing, 9*(1), 83–90.	17-item CMFS was used to examine self-reported fears and anxiety of hospitalized children.	*Sample size*: 82 children. *Sample characteristics*: 8 to 11 years of age, normal cognitive ability, admitted to a pediatric unit for 2–3 days.	*Internal consistency*: Cronbach's alpha = .93 for total CMFS	*Criterion validity*: Significant correlations were found between the total CMSF score and 4 subscale CMFS scores and the STAIC (anxiety) score, .33—.53 ($p < .01$)

TABLE 13.1 *(continued)*

Study citation	CMFS version	Sample and characteristics	Reliability evidence	Validity evidence
Bossart & Hart (1994) *(continued)*				*Discriminant validity:* No significant difference in boys' and girls' fear scores.
Bournaki, M. (1997). Correlates of pain-related responses to venipunctures in school-age children. *Nursing Research, 46,* 147–154.	The 17-item CMFS was used to measure children's levels of reported fears related to medical personnel and diagnostic or therapeutic procedures during a venipuncture.	*Sample size:* 94 children. *Sample characteristics:* 8 to 12 years of age; Mean age = 10.3 years; 86.2% Caucasian; 54.3% female.	*Internal consistency:* Cronbach's alpha = .87 for total	*Content validity Index:* 78% *Criterion validity:* Fear Survey Schedule correlated with CMFS, .71 ($p < .05$). *Construct validity:* No significant differences between girls and boys. No significant difference in medical fear for those experienced vs. not-experienced with venipuncture.
Wilson, A. H., & Yorker, B. (1997). Fears of medical events among school-age children with emotional disorders, parents, and health care providers. *Issues in Mental Health Nursing, 18*(1), 57–71.	17-item CMFS was used to describe the reports of fears of medical events among school-age children with emotional disorders.	*Sample size:* 30 children, 30 parents, and 30 health care providers. *Sample characteristics:* 6 to 14 years of age.	*Internal consistency:* Cronbach's alpha = .75	*Criterion validity:* Children's scores were lower than in previous studies, and were significantly less than their parents' ratings of child fear as well as those of their health care provider.

TABLE 13.1 *(continued)*

Study citation	CMFS version	Sample and characteristics	Reliability evidence	Validity evidence
Wilson & Yorker (1997) *(continued)*				*Discriminant validity:* Boys reported lower fear scores ($p = .006$) than girls.
Beyer, J. E., & Knott, C. B. (1998). Construct validity estimation for the African-American and Hispanic versions of the Oucher scale. *Journal of Pediatric Nursing, 13,* 20–31.	Revised CMFS: 1. Item pertaining to death was excluded. 2. Items referring to school scored as 0 for "N/A" for children who did not go to day care/ school. 3. Format for the items was changed to a question. 4. Children asked to indicate the amount of their fear.	*Sample size:* 104. *Sample characteristics:* 52 African-American patients and 52 Hispanic children, between 3 and 12 years, all having ambulatory surgery	*Internal consistency:* Cronbach's alpha = .79 for total	*Content validity:* A panel of experts judged the content validity as adequate. *Concurrent validity:* Assessed by obtaining concurrent scores for the CMFS and the Fear Survey Schedule $r = .71$ ($p < 0.05$). *Discriminant validity:* In 3 of 4 groups, correlation between fear and pain was nonsignificant; older Hispanic children relationship was .81 ($p < .007$).

lished masters theses and dissertations. In these studies, children were usually between 5 and 12 years of age. In one study, Beyer and Knott (1998) administered the CMFS to children as young as 3 years of age. In all the studies, the CMFS demonstrated adequate internal consistency reliability. Content validity checks were conducted by researchers when they revised the items or response formats substantially, or translated the CMFS into another language. Criterion validity was assessed in several studies by comparing the CMFS with other fear and anxiety scales, and moderately positive relationships were reported. Discriminant validity was tested in several studies. In two, the investigators were interested in distinguishing between the concepts of fear and pain. The CMFS was found to discriminate adequately. In one study, factor analysis documented two subscales: procedural and environmental fears.

CONCLUSIONS AND RECOMMENDATIONS

The Child Medical Fear Scale has been used in a variety of published research studies, as well as theses and dissertations both in and outside of nursing over the last decade (Broome, 1999). In these studies, the CMFS has consistently demonstrated that it is a reliable and valid measure of children's fears of medical experiences. However, there are many areas yet to study related to these fears. For instance, previous studies have reported inconsistent findings related to the gender differences in children's fears. The CMFS has been used in several international studies; yet, there has been no cross-cultural analysis within any study to date that examined whether cultural differences in fear levels exist. Interestingly, several studies have investigated the role of previous experience with illness and hospitalization and CMFS scores and found no relationship. This seems counterintuitive and should be further tested in future studies so that over time this finding can be corroborated and patterns across groups be examined. Another area of interest to nurses should be how children's fears of medical experiences develop over time and whether nursing interventions are effective in reducing high levels of fear that interfere with a child's ability to manage a stressful medical experience. The parent version of the CMFS should be used concurrently when investigating children's fears of medical experiences. Parents' perceptions can give nurses further insight into whether parents should be included in any intervention designed to ameliorate a child's fears.

Although medical fears are only one variable found to influence a child's response to stressful health care experiences (Broome & Huth, 2000), it is an important one and one that has strong clinical utility. The CMFS can help both researchers and clinicians to better understand children and offer them more individualized interventions.

REFERENCES

Abu-Saad, J. J., Pool, M., & Tulkens, B. (1994). Further validity testing of the Abu-Saad Paediatric Pain Assessment Tool. *Journal of Advanced Nursing, 19,* 1063–1071.

Beyer, J. E., & Knott, C. B. (1998). Construct validity estimation for the African-American and Hispanic versions of the Oucher scale. *Journal of Pediatric Nursing, 13,* 20–31.

Bournaki, M. (1997). Correlates of pain-related responses to venipunctures in school-age children. *Nursing Research, 46,* 147–154.

Broome, M. (1999). *Manual for the child medical fear scale.* University of Alabama at Birmingham. broomem@son.uab.edu

Broome, M. E., Bates, T. A., Lillis, P. P., & McGahee, T. W. (1992). Children's medical fears, coping behaviors, and pain perceptions during a lumbar puncture. *Oncology Nursing Forum, 17,* 361–367.

Broome, M. E., Hellier, A., Wilson, T., Dale, S., & Glanville, C. (1988). Measuring children's fear of medical experiences. In C. F. Waltz & O. L. Strickland (Eds.), *Measurement of nursing outcomes: Vol: Measuring client outcomes.* (pp. 201–214). New York: Springer Publishing.

Broome, M., & Huth, M. (2000). Preparation for hospitalization, surgery and procedures. In M. Craft-Rosenberg & J. Denehy (Eds.). *Nursing interventions for children and their families* (pp. 281–298). Beverly Hills, CA: Sage.

Chaiyawat, W. (2000). *Psychometric properties of the Thai versions of STAIC-R and CMFS-R in Thai school age children.* Unpublished doctoral dissertation, Chulalongkorn University, Bangkok, Thailand. wchaiyawat@hotmail.com

Freud, S. (1865). *A general introduction to psycho-analysis.* (J. Riviere, Trans. & Ed.). New York: Liveright, 1935.

Hart, D., & Bossert, E. (1994). Self-reported fears of hospitalized school-age children. *Journal of Pediatric Nursing, 9*(1), 83–90.

Lerner, R. M. (1997). *Concepts and theories of human development* (3rd ed.). New York: Random House.

Melnyk, B. (1994). Coping with unplanned childhood hospitalization: Effects of information on children and their mothers. *Nursing Research, 43,* 50–55.

Nicastro, E., & Whetsell, M. (1999). Children's fears. *Journal of Pediatric Nursing, 14,* 392–402.

Piaget, J. (1967). *Six psychological studies* (A. Tenzer & D. Elkin, Trans.). New York: Random House. (Original work published 1896)

Steward, M. T., & Steward, D.(1981). Children's conceptions of medical procedures. In R. Bibace & M. Walsh (Eds.). *Children's conceptions of health, illness and bodily function.* (pp. 67–84). San Francisco: Jossey-Bass.

Thompson, R. (1985). *Psychosocial research on pediatric hospitalization and health care.* Springfield, IL: Charles C. Thomas.

Vernon, D. T., Foley, J. M., Sipowitz, R., & Schulman, T. (1965). *The psychological responses of children in hospitalization and illness.* Springfield, IL: Charles C. Thomas.

Wilson, A. H., & Yorker, B. (1997). Fears of medical events among school-age children with emotional disorders, parents, and health care providers. *Issues in Mental Health Nursing, 18(1),* 57–71.

Witkin, H. A. (1974). *Psychological differentiation: studies in development.* New York: Erlbaum.

APPENDIX: CHILDREN'S MEDICAL FEAR SCALE

DIRECTIONS TO CHILD: I am going to ask you some questions about things that you may think about when you are sick, see a doctor, or go to the hospital. I want you to tell me how afraid you are of each of the sentences I read to you. For instance if I say, "I am afraid of throwing up if I am sick." I want you to tell me if you are not at all afraid, a little afraid, or a lot afraid of throwing up when you are sick. Okay? Do you have any questions before we begin?

Not at all A little A lot

1. I am afraid of hurting myself.
2. I am afraid of going to the doctor's office.
3. I am afraid of getting a shot.
4. I am afraid of seeing blood come out of me.
5. I am afraid of going to the hospital.
6. I am afraid of having my finger stuck.
7. I am afraid the doctor and nurse will not tell me what they are going to do to me.
8. I am afraid to throw up.
9. I am afraid of missing school if I'm sick.
10. I am afraid of what I will say when I get hurt.
11. I am afraid if I went to the hospital I would have to stay a long time.
2. I am afraid my friends/family will catch something I have if I'm sick and play with them.
13. I am afraid I might die if I go to the hospital.
14. I am afraid of having the doctor or nurse look down my throat.
15. I am afraid the nurse or doctor will tell me something is wrong with me.
16. I am afraid of being away from my family if I go to the hospital.
17. I am afraid of the doctor or nurse putting a tongue blade in my mouth.

14

The Revised Perception of Empathy Inventory

Kathleen Wheeler

This chapter presents the Revised Perception of Empathy Inventory (PEI), a measure of the client's perception of the nurse's empathy.

PURPOSE

The Revised Perception of Empathy Inventory (PEI) measures the client's perception of the nurse's empathy, and is considered the most accurate, conceptually valid measure of empathy in terms of a health outcome. Empathy is a process that is hierarchical in nature. In the empathic process, the person must perceive the other person's feeling within an interaction, then communicate this perception to the other person, and, finally, the recipient of empathy must perceive understanding from the caregiver. The focus of measurement of this tool is this end stage in the process of empathy: the person's perception as the recipient of empathy (Wheeler, 1990). Even if a nurse has high scores on an empathic personality test, it is the client's perception that is crucial for received empathy to occur. The PEI was designed for use in the hospital setting but can be used in outpatient settings as well by cognitively intact adults where there is a nurse–client relationship. This relationship may be crucial in influencing people to maintain healthy patterns of behavior, promote adherence to treatment, and prevent future illness or relapse.

CONCEPTUAL BASIS

Empathy was defined "as a process of understanding whereby the nurse enters the client's perceptual world, the patient perceives this understanding and confirmation of self occurs as part of this process" (Wheeler, 1990, p. 192). Empathy is a complex and methodologically elusive concept with several phases. The process-oriented nature of this concept

207

has been delineated with each phase thought to measure slightly different constructs, and thus each phase needs a different tool to fulfill validity requirements. The phases of empathy have been delineated by Barrett-Lennard (1981).

Phase 1 empathy reflects the individual's empathic potential and is most accurately measured as a personality disposition or ability of the person possessing the empathy. Layton's (1979) Empathy Test is a nursing tool designed to measure this dimension. (See Wheeler (1990) for an in-depth discussion of empathy measures and their use in nursing.) Phase 2 is empathy expressed and is measured by an observer using a rating scale upon observing the subject's behaviors. Clay's (1984) Empathic Interaction Schedule is an example of this type of tool and has been used to teach empathic interactions in the classroom.

Phase 3 of the empathic process reflects empathy received as an experienced emotion. The individual who is the recipient of empathy within a context such as a provider and patient interaction, most accurately perceives and can best rate it. In fact, empathy as rated by teachers or peers has often been found to be unrelated to that experienced by the patients. One study concludes that only the patients' rating of therapist empathy correlated with outcomes measures, while therapists' and supervisors' ratings of the same sessions did not agree with patient perception and did not predict patient outcome (Freemon, Negrete, Davis, & Korsch, 1971). The PEI is a measure of Phase 3 empathy.

Squier's (1990) model of empathic communication addresses theoretical relationships among a practitioner's empathic understanding, a patient's knowledge of his or her illness and motivation to get better, adherence to treatment advice, and health outcome. In this model, the practitioner's empathy leads to a better understanding of the patient's health problems through more open communication and patient self-disclosure. This allows patients to attain greater knowledge about how to improve their health status and thus promotes adherence to treatment and better health outcomes. In this process, patients are able to share emotional concerns, reduce stress factors in illness, and experience greater satisfaction with health care and enhanced motivation to get well. Squier posits that the essence of good practitioner–patient relationships lies in the presence of empathy and that this is integral to positive health outcomes.

PROCEDURES FOR DEVELOPMENT

The PEI was originally developed as a 33–item scale designed to measure a patient's perception of nurse's empathy (Wheeler, 1990). The empathy subscale of the Barrett Lennard Relationship Inventory (BLRI), consisting of 16 items, is a widely used tool to measure the patient's perception of the therapist empathy (Barrett-Lennard, 1962). The BLRI empathy subscale was revised for the PEI. Although this tool had been used in nursing studies to measure patient perception of nurse empathy, eight of the sixteen items had been identified in the nursing literature as problematic or not relevant to the nurse–patient relationship. For the PEI, these items were deleted. A review of the nursing literature also generated a list of critical attributes of empathy in nursing and nine items that reflected these were prepared and included in the PEI.

In addition, confirmation was identified in the literature as integral to Phase 3 empathy; that is, empathy confirms the patient's sense of self and validates self worth. Jourard (1968) has said that confirmation of the self is having one's feelings, and thus one's existence, acknowledged by another. Critical attributes of confirmation were generated from a qualitative study where patients were asked what caregiver behaviors they experienced as confirming themselves as persons (Drew, 1986). Those items theoretically consistent with empathy were included in the PEI.

Four nurse experts provided content validation of the PEI, and the index of content validity (CVI) was calculated. This is the proportion of items given a rating of quite/very relevant. Three items were deleted because they were rated as not or only somewhat relevant. The CVI was then 35/35 or 1.00. Four patients were asked to assess the tool for face validity and two additional items were deleted. Other items were subsequently deleted after a study of their factor analytic structure was conducted (Wheeler, 1995).

DESCRIPTION

This scale reflects how certain the patient feels about an item being either true or false. A Likert-type scale, ranging from 1 to 4, was used with two grades of yes (very true and moderately true) and two grades of no (somewhat true and not at all true). A 1–4 scale was used in lieu of a 1–6 scale out of concern that patients with significant illness may find it easier to choose the most appropriate answer with a simpler rating scale. Several patients who examined the PEI for face validity had difficulty with discriminating answers on the 1–6 scale.

Two subscales were developed: connectedness and confirmation. The final version of the PEI contains 20 items. Negative items were also included, and positive and negative items were arranged in random fashion, avoiding sequences that might result in a response set.

There are 9 items on the confirmation scale and these are #1, 3, 5, 11, 13, 15, 16, 18, and 19. The 11 items on the connectedness scale include #2, 4, 6, 7, 8, 9, 10, 12, 14, 17, and 20 (see Appendix).

ADMINISTRATION AND SCORING

In order to score, negative items are reversed so that the higher the score, the more empathic the nurse is perceived to be by the patient. The negative items include items #4 and #15. The possible range of scores is 20–80 with a score of 20 representing a totally unempathic perception and a score of 80 representing a totally empathic perception. Individual scores for each subscales may also be calculated.

RELIABILITY AND VALIDITY EVIDENCE

Three studies have been conducted that provide psychometric information for the PEI. Wheeler reported study #1 in 1990. Reliability and validity testing was accomplished with 81 inpatient subjects with the first version of the PEI (Wheeler, 1990). One hypothesis was tested for construct validity. It was hypothesized that there would be an inverse relationship between patient's rating of nurse empathy and patient state anxiety. Pre- and postshift patient anxiety measures were obtained on 22 of the 81 patients using the Spielberger State Inventory (Spielberger, 1983). A significant relationship was found between total empathy scores assigned to the nurse and reduction in patient anxiety ($r = -.52$, $p = .008$). The confirmation of this hypothesis demonstrated construct validity for the PEI. Reliability was supported by a Cronbach's alpha of 0.94. In addition, item-to-total correlations were calculated for each item. Items with item-to-total correlations below .30 were deleted.

Study #2 further supported the construct validity of the PEI. Three measures of empathy with each representing a different phase in the empathic process, were assessed for congruence. Again patient anxiety changes were measured and an inverse relationship between PEI scores and anxiety was hypothesized. Subjects included 30 nursing students and 30 nursing home residents. The residents were asked to rate their student nurse's empathy using the PEI and were also given the Spielberger state anxiety scale before and after the student's clinical rotation. Results support Squirer's model of empathy in that PEI scores moderately and positively correlated to changes in client state anxiety ($r = .45$) in the direction hypothesized.

The congruence between the empathy measures yielded results that support Barrett-Lennard's theoretical speculations regarding different conceptual phases of empathy. Phase 1 empathy, student empathy ability, was assessed with Layton's Empathy Test (Layton, 1979). Phase 2 empathy, instructor rating of student empathy, was measured by a visual analog scale, which consisted of three bipolar statements rating student empathy on a 100mm scale. Phase 3 empathy, the patient perception of the student's empathy, was measured by the PEI. The PEI did not correlate with either the Empathy Test of ability or the instructor rating of student empathy. The Empathy Test did correlate significantly with the instructor evaluation of student empathy $r = .26$). All correlations were at the .05 level. However, the Empathy Test's reliability was found to be quite low, at 0.40, for this sample so that correlations with the Empathy Test are suspect.

Cronbach's alpha for the PEI was .96 for this sample. Subjects reported difficulty with the negatively worded items, so these were reworded to reflect positive statements and the revised form included only two randomly placed negatively worded items. Several other items identified as problematic were reworded.

Study #3 employed factor analytic procedures in order to confirm reliability as well as to assess the factor structure of the PEI (Wheeler, 1995). It was expected that two factors would be present: empathy and confirmation. Data from studies #1 and #2 were pooled along with further respondents drawn from an inpatient hospital setting. A total of 151 respondents was obtained. A principal components factor analysis was conducted. Seven factors with eigenvalues >1.0 accounted for 77% of the variance. The first two factors were particularly strong. All confirmation items loaded on factor 1, accounting for 44% of the variance, nine items loaded on factor 2, accounting for 10% of the variance, and this was referred to as the connectedness factor. The most salient dimension of empathy, confirmation, which accounted for 44% of the variability, included items such as "feel confident," "feel energetic," "gives strength," "feel relaxed," and "instills hope." All of these items suggest enhanced physiological well-being for the subject based on the nurse–patient encounter. Thus the factor analysis tended to confirm the factor structure of the PEI. Coefficient theta was also calculated based on the factor solution. These coefficients for the two factors were found to be 0.94 and 0.92, respectively. Those items with low discrimination were deleted and 20 items now remain on the PEI.

CONCLUSIONS AND RECOMMENDATIONS

The Revised Perception of Empathy Inventory demonstrates good reliability in several studies ranging from .92 to .96. It is recommended, however, that additional reliability analysis be conducted for all samples whenever using this tool. It is important to be careful when interpreting scores of subjects from different cultures or language backgrounds.

Although several researchers have asked to use this tool in their research, results have not been reported to the author. The studies reported here demonstrate acceptable reliability and content and construct validity. Further validation of the two-factor structure of the PEI is warranted.

Future studies are important in order to link empathy with health outcome. Outcomes such as severity of symptoms, pain perception, stress-related illnesses, adherence to treatment, prevention, and self-care strategies could be measured for a possible relationship with the PEI. Demonstrating a relationship between the patient's perception of nurse empathy and salubrious health outcomes would further validate the model upon which the PEI is based, thus strengthening evidence for construct validity.

There are a number of other areas that point to further investigation. One area is the assessment of the psychometric properties of the PEI in various settings. For example, the mean scores of the PEI in a nursing home setting could vary from those of the inpatient groups. The setting itself may influence patient receptivity to empathy, and therefore the psychometric properties of the PEI. In a short-term emergency or crisis situation, empathy may be less important than for chronic, long-term illnesses where relationships are thought to be particularly crucial. This proposition has been supported in the nursing literature (Morse, et. al.,1992; Tyner, 1985; Welch-McCaffrey, 1884).

Limitations of the above studies include the use of convenience sampling and inability to replicate the studies. The initial evidence of reliability and validity for the PEI is encouraging, but additional research is needed using diverse samples. The findings from these studies suggest that the PFI can be used with confidence.as an outcome measure for nursing practice.

REFERENCES

Barrett-Lennard, G. T. (1962). Dimension of therapist response as causal factors in therapist change. *Psychological Monographs, 76*(43, Whole No. 562).

Barrett-Lennard, G. T. (1981). The empathy cycle: Refinement of a nuclear concept. *Journal of Counseling Psychology, 28,* 91–100.

Clay, M. (1984). Development of an empathic interaction skills schedule in a nursing context. *Journal of Advanced Nursing, 9,* 343–350.

Drew, N. (1986). Exclusion and confirmation: A phenomenology of patients' experiences with caregivers. *Image: The Journal of Nursing Scholarship, 18,* 39–43.

Freemon, B., Negrete, V. F., Davis, M., and Korsch, B. M. (1971). Gaps in doctor–patient communication: Doctor–patient interaction analysis. *Pediatric Research, 5,* 298–311.

Jourard, S. (1968). *Disclosing man to himself.* New York: Van Nostrand.

Layton, J. M. (1979). Empathy Test—Forms I and II. In M. J. Ward & M. Fetler (Eds.), *Instruments for use in nursing education research.* (pp. 152–

160). Denver, CO: Western Interstate Commission for Higher Education.

Morse, J. M., Anderson, G., Bottoroff, O. Y., O'Brien, B., Solberg, S. M., and Hunter Mellveen, K. M. (1992). Exploring empathy: A conceptual fit for nursing practice? *Image: The Journal of Nursing Scholarship, 24*(4), 273–280.

Spielberger, C. D. (1983). *Manual for the State-Trait Anxiety Inventory.* Palo Alto, CA: Consulting Psychologist Press.

Squier, R. W. (1990). A model of empathic understanding and adherence to treatment regimens in practitioner–patient relationships. *Social Science Medicine, 30*(3), 325–339.

Tyner, R. (1985). Elements of empathic care for dying patients and their families. *Nursing Clinics of North America, 20,* 393–401.

Welch-McCaffrey, D. (1984). Promoting the empathic development of nursing students in the care of the patient with cancer. *Journal of Nursing Education, 23,* 73–76.

Wheeler, K. (1990). Perception of empathy inventory. In O. L. Strickland & C. F. Waltz (Eds.), *Measurement of nursing outcomes: Vol. 4: Measuring client self-care and coping skills* (pp. 181–198). New York: Springer Publishing Co.

Wheeler, K. (1995). Development of the Perception of Empathy Inventory. *International Journal of Psychiatric Nursing Research, 1*(3), 82–88.

APPENDIX: REVISED PERCEPTION OF EMPATHY INVENTORY

Below are listed many different ways that you might feel about your nurse. Please circle the number to the right of each statement that best describes how you feel.

	NOT AT ALL TRUE	SOMEWHAT TRUE	MODERATELY TRUE	VERY TRUE
1. I feel more confident about myself when she/he takes care of me	1	2	3	4
2. She/he knows how to place her/himself in my shoes	1	2	3	4
3. 1 feel more energetic when she/he takes care of me	1	2	3	4
4. Sometimes she/he does not know what I mean	1	2	3	4
5. She/he gives me strength	1	2	3	4
6. She/he makes me feel worthwhile	1	2	3	4
7. 1 can make decisions easier because of her/him	1	2	3	4
8. She/he seems to be involved with my care	1	2	3	4
9. She/he understands me	1	2	3	4
10. 1 feel she/he respects me	1	2	3	4
11. She/he instills hope in me	1	2	3	4
12. 1 feel she/he is in touch and connected with me when she/he takes care of me	1	2	3	4
13. She/he makes me feel more relaxed	1	2	3	4
14. She/he accepts me as I am	1	2	3	4
15. Sometimes I have difficulty communicating with her/him	1	2	3	4
16. When she/he is taking care of me I do not feel so alone	1	2	3	4
17. When I do not say what I mean at all clearly, she/he still understands me	1	2	3	4
18. 1 feel comforted just being with her/him	1	2	3	4
19. Even when she/he is silent I know she/he understands	1	2	3	4
20. She/he cares about me and is genuinely concerned about my welfare	1	2	3	4

For permission to use or reproduce this test, contact Dr. Kathleen Wheeler at Fairfield University, School of Nursing, Fairfield, Connecticut 06430.

PART III
Measuring Care and Quality of Care

15

Measuring Patient Satisfaction with Nursing Care

Lillian R. Eriksen

This chapter discusses the revision of the Patient Satisfaction with Nursing Care scale, a measure of patient satisfaction with nursing care in the hospital setting.

PURPOSE

The purpose of the Revised Patient Satisfaction with Nursing Care instrument is to measure patient satisfaction with nursing care in the hospital setting using a Likert scaling model. The original instrument used a magnitude estimation scaling model (see Eriksen, 1988). The objective of the revised version was to develop a reliable and valid measure that is simpler to use than the previous magnitude estimation scaling model.

CONCEPTUAL BASIS

As with the original instrument, Donabedian's (1980) view that patient satisfaction represents the patient's judgment on the quality of care was used as the base for proceeding with a concept analysis of patient satisfaction. Donabedian also noted that the patient's judgment is based on how well the health care provider meets the expectations and values of the patient. As a result of a concept analysis, patient satisfaction with nursing care was defined as "the patient's subjective evaluation of the cognitive/emotional response that results from the interaction of the patient's expectations of nursing care and the patient's perceptions of actual nurse behaviors and characteristics" (Eriksen, 1995, p. 71).

The conceptual framework of Ware (Ware & Snyder, 1975), used in the original instrument development, was replaced with one developed by Cottle (1989) and refined by Parasuraman, Berry, and Zeithaml (1991). This framework included the dimensions of reliability, assurance, tangibles, responsiveness, and empathy. One dimension was added, 'information giving,' to reflect the role of nurses in educating and informing patients. The identified critical attributes resulting from the concept analysis work were used to examine the existing instrument and to develop new items for the revised instrument. Existing items and new items were examined for their applicability to the definition and framework, resulting in a 34-item instrument representing the six dimensions (Eriksen, 1995).

PROCEDURES FOR DEVELOPMENT

The 34-item instrument used a norm-referenced measurement framework and a Likert-type scaling model with a range of 0 to 6. For purposes of testing reliability and validity of the instrument the 34 items were randomly distributed on the questionnaire and the rating scale was described as: 0 = *expectations not met at all,* 1 = *a lot less than expected,* 2 = *a little less than expected,* 3 = *as expected,* 4 = *exceeded expectations a little,* 5 = *exceeded expectations a lot,* 6 = *way beyond expectations.* Items were formulated in terms of nurse characteristics or behaviors likely to be experienced by patients in the hospital setting.

SCORING AND ADMINISTRATION

The instrument is in the form of a self-administered questionnaire (See Appendix). Subsequent to the testing reported below, the instrument has 12 items organized into two factors. The factors represent two subscales: 'Art of Care' and 'Tangibles/Environment.' Results of the reliability and validity testing support the use of mean scores from each factor or the total scale to get a mean total satisfaction score.

RELIABILITY AND VALIDITY

One large urban hospital and two medium-sized urban hospitals were used as the setting for the two-stage testing of the reliability and validity of this revised patient satisfaction with nursing care instrument. One large urban hospital was used for the first stage and the two medium sized hospitals were used for the second stage.

Patients were contacted the day of discharge to participate in the study. All respondents were hospitalized a minimum of three days on the unit of discharge; oriented to person, place, and time; at least 21 years of age; and capable of reading English. Demographic variables collected regarding the respondents included age, sex, length of hospital stay, length of stay on unit of discharge, number of times previously hospitalized in current hospital, and number of times hospitalized in other hospitals.

Nursing personnel identified eligible participants from their knowledge of patients being discharged. The purposes of the study and an estimate of the time required to complete the questionnaire were read to the potential participant and confidentiality of responses was assured. If the potential participant was willing to participate, the written directions were reviewed and any questions the respondent initiated were answered. An addressed envelope that could be sealed and the questionnaire were left with each willing participant. The investigator returned to each respondent's room to retrieve the questionnaires.

Initial testing for reliability focused on item analyses, including correlations of item to item, item to subscale score, and item to total score. The intraclass correlation coefficient (ICC) was calculated for each subscale and for the total scale.

Construct validity testing was done first with an exploratory factor analysis using SPSS. Principal axis factoring with a varimax rotation revealed a two-factor solution. The software program EQS was used to identify a model that would fit the responses from the first set of data starting with the two-factor solution that emerged from the exploratory factor analysis. This model was then tested on the second set of data to confirm the structure of the instrument. Predictive validity was tested by asking nurse managers in the settings which units would have the highest patient satisfaction scores and which the lowest.

The respondent sample for the first stage included a total of 230 patients from one large urban hospital. The sample used for the second stage of testing included 103 patients from the two medium-sized hospitals.

The first-stage exploratory factor analysis using principal axis factoring with a varimax rotation revealed two distinct factors with eigenvalues greater than one, rather than the six expected from the identified framework. The two factors were labeled "Art of Care" and "Tangibles/Environment." These two factors with distinct and strong associations between the factor and each of its indicants explained 64.2% of the variance (see Table 15.1).

The resultant two-factor solution with 16 items was then examined using a structural equation modeling program (EQS). At this point the Comparative Fit Index (CFI) noted by Bentler (1988) was used to test the model fit to avoid an underestimation of a model fit when dealing with small samples. The results indicated that the model could be further refined as the Comparative Fit Index was 0.87, which was below 0.90 recommended by Bentler. The standardized residuals were examined and those items with the highest residuals were reviewed for removal from the instrument. The items dropped from the Art of Care scale were 'attention,' and 'unhurried.' The items 'smell' and 'uniform' were dropped

TABLE 15.1 Factor Structure Resulting From the Principal Axis Factoring With Varimax Rotation

Art of care		Tangibles/environment	
Attention of nurses	.76	Grooming of nurses	.75
Patience of nurses	.75	Things done on time	.73
In good hands	.75	Explained how to help self	.72
Clear information	.75	Room neat & orderly	.71
Courtesy of nurses	.75	Appearance of uniform	.71
Unhurried approach	.71	Nurses smell clean	.71
Got help when needed	.70	Oriented to room & hospital	.66
Explained tests & procedures	.63	Controlled noise	.49

from the Tangibles/Environment scale because they were both represented by the more general item 'grooming.' Thus a total of 12 items remained in the instrument. The repeated testing of the CFI was .98 indicating a very good fit of the data to the structured model (see Figure 15.1).

The model was then tested for the presence of a higher-order factor, namely 'Patient Satisfaction.' The structure of the proposed model is presented in Figure 15.2. The CFI for this model was .991, indicating an improvement in fit and that a higher-order factor better explained the data and made substantive sense.

The second stage of testing of the instrument was a confirmatory analysis to investigate if the model developed in the first stage would be confirmed with the second set of data from the two medium-sized hospitals. As hypothesized, the model was confirmed as structured in the results of the first stage of testing and refinement. The CFI for this second data set was .95.

Internal consistency reliability was tested using the Intra Class Correlation Coefficient (ICC). Each subscale and the total scale were estimated separately for each stage of testing in the two samples. The results presented in Table 15.2 reveal consistently high reliabilities.

TABLE 15.2 ICC Reliability Estimates for Both Test Times Including 95% Confidence Intervals

Testing	Art of care subscale	Tang./environ. subscale	Total scale
Sample 1	.93 (.91–.94)	.88 (.85–.91)	.94 (.92–.95)
Sample 2	.93 (.91–.95)	.93 (.90–.95)	.96 (.94–.97)

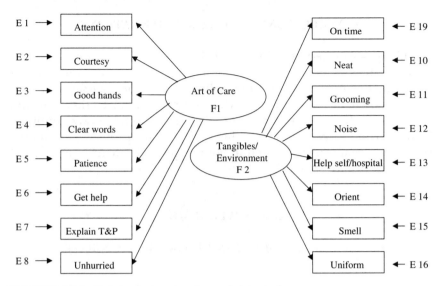

FIGURE 15.1 Original structural model tested.

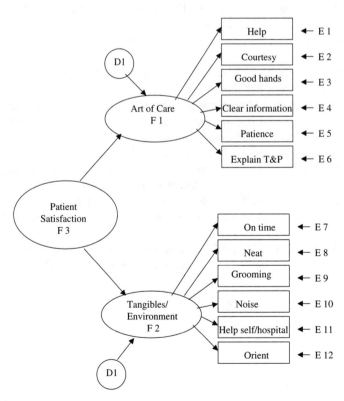

FIGURE 15.2 Model of higher order factor structure.

CONCLUSIONS AND RECOMMENDATIONS

This two-stage testing of this revised measure of patient satisfaction with nursing care in the hospital setting represents a revision based on conceptual analysis work and tested first with factor analyses leading to the development and testing of a measurement model using structural equation modeling techniques. The measurement model was confirmed in the second stage of testing using a second set of data. The internal consistency reliability was tested in both stages and revealed high reliability results in both stages.

ACKNOWLEDGMENT

This research was supported by NINR Fellowship F32 NR06603.

REFERENCES

Bentler, P. M. (1988). Comparative fit indexes in structural models. *Psychological Bulletin, 107,* 238–246.
Cottle, D. W. (1989). *Client-centered service: How to keep them coming back for more.* New York: Wiley.
Donabedian, A. (1980). *The definition of quality and approaches to its measurement.* Ann Arbor, MI: Health Administration Press.
Eriksen, L. R. (1988). Measuring patient satisfaction with nursing care: A magnitude estimation approach. In C. F. Waltz & O. L. Strickland (Eds), *Measurement of nursing outcomes: Vol. 1: Measuring client outcomes* (pp. 523–537). New York: Springer Publishing Co.
Eriksen, L. R. (1995). Patient satisfaction with nursing care: Concept clarification. *Journal of Nursing Measurement, 3*(4), 59–76.
Parasuraman, A., Berry, L. L., & Zeithaml, V. A. (1991). Understanding customer expectations of service. *Sloan Management Review, 32*(3), 39–46.
Ware, J., Jr., & Snyder, M. (1975). Dimensions of patient attitudes regarding doctors and medical care services. *Medical Care, 13,* 669–682.

APPENDIX: PATIENT SATISFACTION WITH NURSING CARE INDEX

Please help us improve our nursing care by completing this questionnaire.

This questionnaire is to be answered by the patient receiving nursing care. It is OK to assist the patient in writing the answers but the responses should be those of the **patient.**

Everyone has some idea of what they expect of the nurses taking care of them. Listed below are some characteristics or behaviors of nurses which patients have said influence their satisfaction with nursing care.

Think about **your expectations** of nursing care. As you read each item on the questionnaire decide to what **degree your experience** with nursing care **on this unit** did or did not meet your **expectations.** There are not any right or wrong answers, only your opinion. The numbers 0 to 6 indicate the degree to which Your **expectations were met.**

> 0 - Expectations not met at all
> 1 - lot less than expected
> 2 - A little less than expected
> 3 - As expected
> 4 - Exceeded expectations a little
> 5 - Exceeded expectations a lot
> 6 - Way beyond expectations

My age is _____ years. I am _____ Female _____ Male
I have been a patient at this hospital _____ other times beside this time.
I have been a patient in other hospitals _____ times.
I have been in the hospital this time about _____ days.

	Not met at all	Lot less than expected	Little less than expected	As expected	Exceeded a little	Exceeded a lot	Way beyond expectations
1. Getting help with things I couldn't do for myself.	0	1	2	3	4	5	6
2. Courtesy of my nurses.	0	1	2	3	4	5	6
3. Feeling like I was in "in good hands" with my nurses.	0	1	2	3	4	5	6
4. When explaining things nurses use words I understand.	0	1	2	3	4	5	6
5. Patience of my nurses.	0	1	2	3	4	5	6
6. Explaining tests and procedures so I could understand what would happen to me during the test or procedure.	0	1	2	3	4	5	6

	Not met at all	Lot less than expected	Little less than expected	As expected	Exceeded a little	Exceeded a lot	Way beyond expectations
7. Nurses kept my room neat and orderly.	0	1	2	3	4	5	6
8. The grooming of my nurses.	0	1	2	3	4	5	6
9. Nurses gave me my medicines and treatments on time.	0	1	2	3	4	5	6
10. Nurses controlled the noise in my room	0	1	2	3	4	5	6
11. Nurses told me what to do for myself while in the hospital	0	1	2	3	4	5	6
12. Nurses oriented me to my room.	0	1	2	3	4	5	6

On a scale of 1 to 10, with **1** the **lowest** and **10** the **highest,** I would rate my overall satisfaction with my nursing care as a _____.

If there are any other comments you would like to make please feel free to write them on the back of the page. Thank you for your assistance.

16

Measure of Patient Satisfaction with Nursing Care: Spanish Language Translation

Lillian R. Eriksen and Judi Witter

This chapter discusses the Spanish language translation of the Patient Satisfaction with Nursing Care Instrument, a measure of patient satisfaction with nursing care in the hospital setting.

PURPOSE

The multicultural environment in which health care is delivered challenges the measurement of outcomes in health care research. Instruments to measure outcomes in populations that include participants who do not read and write English require translation into the language of the participants. Measurement of patient satisfaction as an outcome of nursing care has generally been limited to English literate participants. Estimates of the population of Hispanics residing in the United States by the year 2020 range from 47 million to 54 million (Marin & Marin, 1991). The increase in the size of the Hispanic population in the United States requires the availability of instruments to measure outcomes in this enlarging segment of our population. This became evident when a number of patient responses on the English version of an instrument to measure patient satisfaction with nursing care were written in Spanish.

The purpose of this study was to develop an equivalent Spanish language translation of an existing English language instrument to measure patient satisfaction with nursing care in the hospital setting. The translation processes and the equivalence testing of the instrument are presented.

PROCEDURES FOR DEVELOPMENT

Translation of instruments requires a cultural understanding of not only the content but also the context and style of the culture receiving the translation (Werner & Campbell, 1973). Two differing types of translation approaches can be used, depending on the goal of the translation work. The symmetrical or decentered method strives for equality of meaning and colloquialness in both languages (Werner & Campbell, 1973). This approach is also recommended when a goal is to make comparisons or reference the concept across cultures (Chapman & Carter, 1979) The second type of translation is the assymetrical or unicentered approach. The assymetrical method emphasizes loyalty to one of the languages used, usually the original language of the work being translated (Werner & Campbell, 1973).

Because the aim of this translation work was equivalence of both an English and Spanish version of an instrument for measuring patient satisfaction, the symmetrical or decentered approach was used. The symmetrical approach allows a more culturally appropriate instrument that would encourage participation of Hispanic patients in the evaluation of their satisfaction with nursing care. The decentering method is an iterative process involving translation from the source language into the target language and then back translation until there is agreed-on meaning for both languages (Brislin, Lonner & Thorndike, 1973). In this approach both languages are respected as equally important, and wording of items is open to modification in both languages as needed.

The first attempt of translation of the satisfaction instrument instructions to respondents and items from English into Spanish was accomplished by three Spanish-speaking nurses working independently. Two of the bilingual nurses were staff nurses and one was a diabetes educator who taught her classes in Spanish. The three nurses then reviewed their work together. This review of the translation revealed significant differences in words and meaning. Subsequently, a professional translator from a local college provided another translation of the instrument. The three Spanish-speaking nurses reviewed the Spanish version of the professional translator. The review confirmed the appropriateness of the professionally translated version.

The Spanish translation was then back translated into English by another bilingual nurse. The back translation was reviewed by the three original nurses for equivalence of meaning in English. Also, the original developer of the instrument reviewed the back translation to assess if it represented the intention of the original instrument. It was agreed that the Spanish and English versions seemed to be equivalent in meaning both to the translators and the original developer of the English version. Once the equivalence of meaning was agreed on, the instruments were field tested to assess their statistical equivalence.

BACKGROUND OF THE ENGLISH VERSION

The patient satisfaction instrument (Eriksen, 1988) was the revised instrument based on subsequent concept analysis work (Eriksen, 1995).

Patient satisfaction with nursing care is defined as the degree to which the patient's expectations of nurses is met. The revised instrument was first tested in two hospitals in the southwestern United States. The revised framework included the concepts of (1) dependability, (2) responsiveness, (3) information giving, (4) empathy, and (5) tangibles. When tested, the proposed factor structure using the five concepts as subscales was not supported. Instead a one-factor solution using items from each of the five concepts resulted in a 15-item questionnaire. (See Appendix for copy of the instrument). At this time the need for a Spanish version of the instrument was identified and the translation process pursued.

EQUIVALENCY TESTING

Bilingual subjects were selected from the population of patients from a large hospital located in the southwestern part of the country. Marín, and Marín (1991) describe two types of bilinguals. The first is the coordinate bilingual who learned the two or more languages at different times and preferably in the cultures represented by the languages. The second is the compound bilingual who learned both languages at the same time. For this study it seemed the coordinate bilingual would be appropriate, as most of the Spanish-speaking population in this hospital had learned Spanish first in a Spanish-speaking culture. Therefore, bilingual patients who had spoken Spanish as their first language and English as a second language were recruited. As the intent of the development of the Spanish version was to enable Spanish-speaking patients to evaluate their satisfaction with nursing care, this would be the appropriate type of bilingual person to test the instrument.

Data Collection and Sample

A sample size of 15 was required for the equivalency testing using Pearson's *r*. This was based on the expectation of a fairly large effect (.70) and a power of .90 (Kramer & Theimann, 1987). The sample consisted of 16 men and 16 women ranging in age from 35 to 86 years. The mean age was 69 with a median of 69 and a mode of 64 years of age. Bilingual respondents were identified, informed of the study, and asked if they would like to participate. The willing participants were given instructions in English by a nurse. On a rotating basis the English and Spanish versions were presented first for completion. Once the first form was completed by the participant the same nurse retrieved it and the other language form was administered. When both forms were completed they were forwarded to the quality assurance department. Thus the sample consisted primarily of older adults with both genders equally represented.

EQUIVALENCY TESTING RESULTS

The mean scores and standard deviations for both versions of the instrument presented in Table 16.1 reveal very similar results for both the English and Spanish versions of the instrument. As hypothesized, the paired samples *t*-test revealed no significant difference between the mean scale scores of the English and Spanish versions ($df = 31$, $t = .14$, $p = .444$). The mean scale score for the English version was 3.07 and for the Spanish version 3.07.

The Pearson correlation between the mean scores on the two versions was .99. Individual item correlations between the English and Spanish versions ranged from .89 to 1.0 (Table 16.2). Item-to-total score correlations for both the English and Spanish versions of the instruments are presented in Table 16.3. A high degree of agreement is evident in the similar patterns of item-to-total score correlations for both language versions. The Cronbach's internal consistency reliability for both versions was .96.

CONCLUSIONS

Equivalence of the Spanish and English versions of the instrument is well supported by the findings of the testing. The similarity of the means and standard deviations of the items in both languages and the nonsignificant finding in differences between mean scale scores support equivalence. In addition the correlations tested revealed a pattern consistent with equivalence. The translation processes and testing indicate that this Spanish version of a measure of patient satisfaction with nursing care is appropriate to use with patients who have learned Spanish as their first language.

TABLE 16.1 Item Scores for English and Spanish Versions

	Mean	SD	Minimum	Maximum
Item 1				
English	2.94	1.05	1	5
Spanish	2.81	1.00	0	5
Item 2				
English	3.06	.84	1	5
Spanish	3.03	.82	1	5
Item 3				
English	3.25	.98	1	5
Spanish	3.30	.99	1	6
Item 4				
English	3.38	1.04	1	6
Spanish	3.38	1.04	1	6
Item 5				
English	2.94	1.05	1	6
Spanish	3.00	.98	1	6

TABLE 16.1 *(continued)*

	Mean	*SD*	Minimum	Maximum
Item 6				
English	3.00	1.08	1	5
Spanish	3.03	1.06	1	5
Item 7				
English	3.09	.96	1	6
Spanish	3.16	.88	2	6
Item 8				
English	3.28	1.02	1	6
Spanish	3.25	1.05	1	6
Item 9				
English	3.03	.97	1	6
Spanish	3.06	1.01	1	6
Item 10				
English	3.29	.94	2	6
Spanish	3.19	1.06	1	6
Item 11				
English	2.94	.98	1	5
Spanish	3.00	.88	1	5
Item 12				
English	2.94	.88	1	5
Spanish	2.94	.95	1	5
Item 13				
English	3.19	.97	1	6
Spanish	3.13	.91	1	5
Item 14				
English	2.94	.98	1	6
Spanish	2.94	.91	1	5
Item 15				
English	2.84	1.10	1	5
Spanish	2.78	1.13	0	5

TABLE 16.2 Pearson's Product Moment
Correlation Coefficient between Individual Items
on the English and Spanish Versions

Item #	*R*	Item #	*r*
1	.89	9	.99
2	.88	10	.98
3	.90	11	.93
4	1.00	12	.96
5	.91	13	.97
6	.99	14	.97
7	.93	15	.96
8	.99		

TABLE 16.3 Item to Total Score Correlation for Spanish and English Versions

Item #	English	Spanish	Item #	English	Spanish
1	.89	.91	9	.84	.82
2	.84	.86	10	.77	.76
3	.88	.84	11	.89	.85
4	.73	.73	12	.86	.87
5	.89	.87	13	.77	.79
6	.91	.88	14	.79	.84
7	.83	.84	15	.81	.85
8	.83	.85			

REFERENCES

Brislin, R. W., Lonner, W. J., & Thorndike, R. M. (1973). *Cross-cultural research methods.* New York: Wiley.

Chapman, D. W., & Carter, J. F. (1979). Translation procedures for the cross-cultural use of measurement. *Educational Evaluation and Policy Analysis, 1*(3), 71–76.

Eriksen, L. R. (1988). Measuring patient satisfaction with nursing care. A magnitude estimation approach. In Strickland, O. L. & Waltz, C. F. (Eds.), *Measurement of nursing outcomes: Vol. 1: Measuring client outcomes.* (pp. 523–534). New York: Springer Publishing Co.

Eriksen, L. R. (1995). Patient satisfaction with nursing care: Concept clarification. *Journal of Nursing Measurement, 3*(1), 59–76.

Kramer, H. C., & Theimann, S. (1987). *How many subjects? Statistical power analysis in research.* Newbury Park: Sage.

Marín, G., & Marín, B. V. (1991) *Research with Hispanic populations.* Newbury Park, CA: Sage.

Werner, O., & Campbell, D. (1973). Translating, working through interpreters and the problem of decentering. In R. Naroll & R. Cohen (Eds.), *American handbook of methods in cultural anthropology* (pp. 398–420). New York: Columbia University Press.

APPENDIX: CENSA DE SATISFACCION PARA LOS PACIENTES

Por favor ayudenos a mejorar el cuidado de enfermeras acompletando este cuestionario.

Cada paciente abe y espera cual es el cuidado de una enfermera. Continuacion encontrara una lista de carateristicas o comportamientos de enfermeras que algunos pacientes han proporcionado que influye a la satisfaccion del cuidado de enfermeras.

Piense sobre lo que Ud. Espera del cuidado de enfermeras. Como Ud. Vaya leyendo cada articulo en el cuestionario, decida a que grado su experiencia con el cuidado de enfermeras en este piso had sido, o no satis fechas. No hay respuestas buenas o males, solo su opinion. Los numeros 0 a 6 indican hasta que grado
sus necesidades fueron satisfechas.

0 - Necesidades no fueron satisfechas
1 - Mucho menos de lo esperado
2 - Un poco menps de lo esperado
3 - Como esperado
4 - Un poco mas de lo esperado
5 - Sufficiente mas de lo esperado
6 - Mucho mas de lo esperado

Si tu eres el PACIENTE, contesta estas preguntas, por favor:

Mi edad es _____. Sexo: _____Feminino _____Masculino

He sido un paciente de (Hospital nombre) antes de esta vez ____si ____no. Cuantas veces ____.

He sido un paciente de otros hospitales ____si ____no. Cuantas veces ____.

Esta visita he estado aqui por ____ dias.

Si usted es FAMILIA/AMIGOS del paciente, favor de contestar estas preguntas del paciente.

Commentar en el otro lado de esta pagina.

	Necesidades no fueron satisfechas	Mucho menos de lo esperado	Un poco menps de lo esperado	Como esperado	Un poco mas de lo esperado	Sufficiente mas de lo esperado	Mucho mas de lo esperado
1. La atencion individual que la enfermera me proprociono.	0	1	2	3	4	5	6

	Necesidades no fueron satisfechas	Mucho menos de lo esperado	Un poco menps de lo esperado	Como esperado	Un poco mas de lo esperado	Sufficiente mas de lo esperado	Mucho mas de lo esperado
2. Recibiendo la ayuda en las cosas que no pude hacer por mi mismo.	0	1	2	3	4	5	6
3. Enfermeras manteniendome informado sobre lo que estaba occurriendo0		1	2	3	4	5	6
4. Recubu la ayuda de una enfermera cuando la necesitaba.	0	1	2	3	4	5	6
5. Cortesia por parte de mis enfermeras.	0	1	2	3	4	5	6
6. Sintiendo que estoy en "buenas manos" con mis enfermeras.	0	1	2	3	4	5	6
7. En caso de alguna explicacion las enfermeras usan palabras que yo puedo entender.	0	1	2	3	4	5	6
8. Compasion por parte de mis enfermeras.	0	1	2	3	4	5	6
9 Explicacion sobre pruebas y procedimientos de una manera que yo puedo entender que me pasara durante la prueba o procedimiento	0	1	2	3	4	5	6
10. Rapidez en contestar la luz/el boton de emergencia/regrecar la llamada por telefono.	0	1	2	3	4	5	6
11. La apariencia profesional en los uniformes de las enfermeras.	0	1	2	3	4	5	6
12. Las enfermeras me hacen sentir seguro.	0	1	2	3	4	5	6
13. La frequencia con que las enfermeras se preocupan por mi y mi condicion	0	1	2	3	4	5	6
14. Las enfermeras ponen de las necicidades de que yo tenga, como las luz de emergencia, aqua, telefono, toallas sanitaria, de un modo que sea para mi facil de obtenerlos.	0	1	2	3	4	5	6
15. Incluyendome a mi en planes y arreglos para mi cuidado.	0	1	2	3	4	5	6

En la escala del 1 al 10, con el numero 1 el mas bajo, y el 10 el mas alto, yo ratificare mi absoluta satisfaccion del cuidado de mi enfermera como:_____.

Si Ud. Tiene algun otro comentario que quiera aportat por favor hagalo en frente de esta paglna.

Gracias por su asistencia.

17

Measuring the Caring Process in Nursing: The Caring Behavior Checklist and the Client Perception of Caring Scale

Anna M. McDaniel

This chapter discusses the Caring Behavior Checklist and the Client Perception of Caring Scale, two measures of caring behaviors of nurses.

PURPOSE

Caring has been traditionally viewed by nurses and the public as the basis for the nursing profession. However, increases in technology and specialization have contributed to the depersonalization of health care in our society today (Carper, 1979). Perhaps in response, current nursing literature has shown an increase in theoretical and scientific exploration of the phenomenon of caring. This study was proposed to develop valid methods for the investigation of the components of the caring process.

CONCEPTUAL BASIS

A dichotomy exists in the definitions of care in nursing. In the ANA Position Paper of 1965 (American Nurses' Association, 1965), nursing is described as caring for and caring about. From a nursing perspective, caring for incorporates the activities involved in taking care of. Much effort in nursing and nursing education is directed toward this aim. Nurses give back care, hygienic care, and catheter care. However, it cannot be assumed from the performance of such caregiving activities that the nurse cares about.

In discussing caring about, nursing authors draw heavily on the existential philosophers Marcel and Buber (Reiman, 1986; Valliot, 1966; Watson, 1985). Caring about involves the sharing of human experiences and existence. It requires that the nurse adopt an attitude of regard for the being of the individual. However, unless this motivates the nurse to act or care for, caring has not actually taken place.

According to Bevis (1981), "caring demands that feelings be converted into behaviors and that the behaviors and feelings be accompanied by thoughts" (p. 50). True caring must encompass both concepts: caring for and caring about. When developing a theoretical definition of caring, one needs to examine the relationship between the philosophical context of caring about and the behavioral context of caring for. This can be accomplished by conceptualizing caring as a process or series of actions intended to achieve a certain result.

Care is the investment of oneself for the benefit of another (person, group, or institution) without regard for personal gain. In nursing, care is the investment of one's personal resources in another in order to promote well-being. The nurse's personal resources may include, but are not limited to, knowledge, expertise, time, and emotional energy.

The process of caring in nursing can be conceptualized in four levels (Figure 17.1). Acknowledgment of the need for care is the first stage. This involves the nurse's awareness of the human experiences of the other. From an existential perspective, this is described as the "I–Thou" relationship (Reiman, 1986; Valliot, 1966). The I–Thou relationship, in contrast to an "I–It" relationship, involves the sharing of experiences with the other person as a human being. One could postulate that the widespread use of the nursing process has encouraged nurses to adopt an objective I–It view of patients, thus hindering nurses' potential to care.

Once the need for care has been recognized in the other, a decision to care is the next phase. The nurse's self-assessment of personal resources

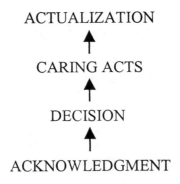

FIGURE 17.1 Conceptual model of the caring process in nursing.

is necessary. The choice to commit these resources to the well-being of the other completes this phase. Gadow (1980) describes this as "unifying and directing of one's entire self in relation to another's need" (p. 90). This involves a willingness by the nurse to risk the cost of caring for the benefit of the other.

The third level in the caring process includes the actions and behaviors of the nurse intended to promote the welfare of the other. As Watson (1985) states, the "essence of the value of human care and caring may be futile unless it contributes to a philosophy of action" (p. 32). Gaut (1984) describes caring as a series of actions. Yet, as Mayeroff (1971) notes, "the process rather than the product is primary in caring" (p. 31). Actions taken on behalf of the other are the external manifestation of the internal cognitive and affective processes of the nurse that have taken place at prior levels.

Actualization of the caring experience is the ultimate result of the caring process. The perception of the other as being cared for and about is the fulfillment of the caring interaction. The realization that caring has occurred promotes growth and satisfaction in both the nurse and the other. Noddings (1984) describes an intangible transformation that takes place in the cared-for and the one caring. Benner (1984) describes this as the transformative power of caring.

PROCEDURES FOR DEVELOPMENT

The purpose of this study was to develop valid methods for the investigation of the components of the caring process. A norm-referenced measurement framework was used to measure caring behaviors and the effect of these actions on the client. The outcome variables of intent were caring behaviors and the client's perception of caring. In this study, caring behaviors were defined as those verbal and nonverbal actions denoting care performed by the nurse. The operational definition of the client's perception of caring was based on the subjective, affective response of the client to the nurse's caring behaviors.

From analysis of current research findings, two tools have been developed to examine the caring process in nursing. The first tool is the Caring Behavior Checklist (see Appendix A). Specific verbal and nonverbal behaviors have been identified a priori as significant indicators of caring (Field, 1984; Gardner & Wheeler, 1981; Larson, 1984; Reiman, 1986; Weiss, 1984). The tool is designed to measure the presence or absence of specific actions denoting care, not to quantify the degree or amount of care.

The second tool, The Client Perception of Caring Scale (see Appendix B), is a questionnaire designed to measure the client's response to the caring behaviors of the nurse. Reiman (1986) suggests that to study "only empirical indicators of caring from the nurse's perspective would not get at the essential structure of the caring interaction as experienced by the client" (p. 86). The items were developed from studies describing the reactions of clients to nurse–client interactions (Field, 1984; Reiman, 1986; Weiss, 1984).

ADMINISTRATION AND SCORING

The two instruments are designed to be used together to measure the caring process. They are intended for use in a hospital setting with patients who have the cognitive skills necessary to complete the instrument. A trained observer scores the Caring Behavior Checklist while observing a nurse–patient interaction for a period of 30 minutes. As noted in Waltz, Strickland, and Lenz (1984), no data should be recorded for the first 10 minutes in order to reduce subject reactivity. Each behavior on the checklist is to be scored dichotomously as present or absent. The checklist consists of 12 items representing the behaviors indicative of caring. The potential range of scores for the instrument is 0 to 12. High scores indicate a high number of behaviors were observed; low scores indicate few behaviors were observed.

The Client Perception of Caring Scale is to be administered to the client following the observation period. The tool consists of 10 items that are rated on a 6–point summated rating scale. Each item value is to be summed to obtain the score. Items 5 and 8 are perceptions associated with noncaring behaviors of the nurse, and the item value is reversed before being summed. The scores for the Client Perception of Caring Scale have a potential range of 10 to 60. High scores indicate a high degree of caring as perceived by the client. Low scores mean that the client perceived low caring behavior in the nurse.

RELIABILITY AND VALIDITY

Both tools have been submitted to two doctorally prepared nurse researchers with experience in the field of caring. The method for determining content validity described in Waltz et al., (1984) was used. The content validity index (CVI) for the Caring Behaviors Checklist was calculated as .80. The CVI for the Client Perception of Caring Scale was determined to be 1.00.

A time sampling of student nurse–patient interactions was used to collect data to determine reliability and validity of the measures. Following approval from the Research Review Committee, a convenience sample of junior-level nursing students from a baccalaureate nursing program was selected. Clients assigned to these participating students for clinical laboratory experience were randomly selected as the client sample. Although students were observed more than once, a total of 21 different student nurse–patient interactions were observed for data collection. Both the students and the clients participating received a verbal explanation of the purpose and procedures of the study before signing a written consent form.

Reliability of the Client Perception of Caring Scale was determined by the internal consistency approach. The standardized item alpha coefficient was calculated at .81. Item-to-total correlation averaged .41 for this scale.

Reliability of the Caring Behavior Checklist was estimated using interrater agreements. Each of the 21 interactions was simultaneously observed by two trained raters, who scored the items independently. The interrater reliability of the Caring Behavior Checklist was determined as a function of agreements between observers. This was calculated by using the following formula: number of agreements divided by total number of agreements and disagreements (Polit & Hungler, 1987). This was first calculated after nine observations and determined at .82. Items 10 and 12 were further clarified, and the raters were given additional instructions. Interrater agreements for the remaining 12 observations was .99. Overall interrater reliability was .92. Interrater reliability for individual items ranged from .76 to 1.00.

The measure used to estimate construct validity of the two caring instruments was the LaMonica Empathy Profile. This tool, formerly known as the LaMonica Empathy Construct Rating Scale, is a 30-item self-report using a forced-choice format. Scores are obtained on five subscales: responding verbally; nonverbal behavior; respect of self and others; openness, honesty, and flexibility; and perceiving feelings and listening. The reliability index for this tool as a self-report was estimated by a coefficient alpha of .96 (LaMonica, 1981). Discriminant validity of this instrument was determined by the multitrait-multimethod approach with $r = .20$ ($p < .001$) (LaMonica, 1981).

A measure of empathy was considered appropriate to estimate construct validity because conceptually it is closely related to caring, and tools measuring the two concepts should be significantly correlated. LaMonica (1981) defines empathy as signifying "a central focus and feeling with and in the client's world by the helper, communication of this understanding to the client, and the client's perception of the helper's understanding" (p. 398). This definition of empathy as a process is similar to the theoretical definition of caring presented here. Empathy is a necessary part of caring, particularly at the acknowledgment level. Indeed, without empathy the caring process would not take place. Noddings (1984) describes the relationship between empathy, feeling with and in, and caring when she states: "Apprehending the other's reality, feeling what he feels as nearly as possible, is the essential part of caring from the view of the one caring. For if I take on the other's reality as possibility and begin to feel its reality, I feel also that I must act accordingly" (p. 16).

To estimate construct validity, the results of the Client Perception of Caring Scale were correlated with the subscale scores on the Empathy Profile. This yielded no significant results at the .05 level. This result could be attributed in part to the low number of subjects or the ipsative nature of the Empathy Profile,which violates the assumptions of independence required for parametric statistics (Kerlinger & Lee, 2000).

As an additional method to evaluate content validity of the Caring Behavior Checklist, each client was asked to respond to the question, "What is the one thing that a nurse does that shows you that he/she really cares about you?" Of the 18 clients responding to this question, 17 identified behaviors that were described in the 12 items on the tool. The one behavior not included on the tool, "Has a soft tone of voice," was identified by a blind client.

CONCLUSIONS AND RECOMMENDATIONS

The analysis of the reliability estimate of the Client Perception of Caring Scale yielded satisfactory results with a standardized alpha coefficient of .81. Because of low item-to-total correlation, revision of item 6 ($r = -.15$) and item 3 ($r = .17$) is indicated. Increasing the length of the scale would result in a higher alpha, for the tool. Although the construct validity assessment in this study did not support the tool's validity, criterion-related validity may be established in replicative studies using a more appropriate instrument, such as the Trusting Relationship Scale of Risser's Patient Satisfaction Instrument as revised by Hinshaw and Atwood (1982), and a larger number of subjects.

By analysis of the interrater reliability of the Caring Behavior Checklist, one can infer that there is agreement between observers when using this tool; that is, the two observers identified the same caring behaviors. Use of this tool as an observation guide to categorize behaviors may be appropriate. However, a limitation of the tool is that the items are dichotomously scored, which reduces score variance. Results obtained from using this tool may be improved by increasing the potential for item variability by weighting items according to patient preferences.

Implications for further study would include observation of a different population of nurses to see if a significant difference in behaviors is found compared to those observed in this study. Prolonging the observation period and standardizing the circumstances of the observation—for example, around specific types of nurse–patient interactions or procedures—may also be indicated.

REFERENCES

American Nurses' Association Committee on Education. (1965). *Educational preparation for nurse practitioners and assistants to nurses: A position paper.* New York: Author.

Benner, P. (1984). *From novice to expert: Excellence and power in clinical nursing practice.* Menlo Park, CA: Addison-Wesley.

Bevis, E. (1981). Caring: A life force. In M. Leininger (Ed.), *Caring: An essential human need* (pp. 49–59). Thorofare, NJ: Charles B. Slack.

Carper, B. (1979). The ethics of caring. *Advances in Nursing Science, 1*(13), 11–19.

Field, P. (1984). Client care-seeking behaviors and nursing care. In M. Leininger (Ed.), *Care: The essence of nursing and health* (pp. 249–262). Thorofare, NJ: Charles B. Slack.

Gadow, S. (1980). Existential advocacy: Philosophical foundations of nursing. In S. Spicker & S. Gadow (Eds.), *Nursing: Images and ideals—opening dialogue with the humanities* (pp. 79–101). New York: Springer.

Gardner, K., & Wheeler, E. (1981). The meaning of caring in the context of nursing. In M. Leininger (Ed.), *Caring: An essential human need* (pp. 69–79). Thorofare, NJ: Charles B. Slack.

Gaut, D. (1984). A theoretical description of caring as action. In M. Leininger (Ed.), *Care: The essence of nursing and health* (pp. 27–44). Thorofare, NJ: Charles B. Slack.

Hinshaw, A., & Atwood, J. (1982). A patient satisfaction instrument: Precision by replication. *Nursing Research, 31,* 170–175.

Kerlinger, F. N., & Lee, H. B. (2000). *Foundations of Behavioral Research* (4th ed.). Fort Worth, TX: Harcourt College Publishers.

LaMonica, E. (1981). Construct validity of an empathy instrument. *Research in Nursing and Health, 4,* 389–400.

Larson, P. (1984). Important nurse caring behaviors perceived by patients with cancer. *Oncology Nursing Forum, 11*(6), 46–50.

Mayeroff, M. (1971). *On caring.* New York: Harper & Row.

McDaniel, A. M. (1990). The caring process in nursing: Two instruments for measuring caring behaviors. In O. Strickland & C. F. Waltz (Eds.), *Measurement of nursing outcomes: Vol. 4: Measuring client self-care and coping skills* (pp. 17–27). New York: Springer Publishing Co.

Noddings, N. (1984). *Caring: A feminine approach to ethics and moral education.* Berkeley, CA: University of California Press.

Polit, D., & Hungler, B. (1987). *Nursing research: Principles and methods* (3rd ed.). Philadelphia: Lippincott.

Reiman, D. (1986). The essential structure of a caring interaction: Doing phenomenology. In P. Munhall & C. Oiler (Eds.), *Nursing research: A qualitative perspective* (pp. 85–106). Norwalk, CT: Appleton-Century-Crofts.

Valliot, M. (1966). Existentialism: A philosophy of commitment. *American Journal of Nursing, 66,* 500–505.

Waltz, C., Strickland, O., & Lenz, E. (1984). *Measurement in nursing research.* Philadelphia: F. A. Davis.

Watson, J. (1985). *Nursing: Human science and human care.* Norwalk, CT: Appleton-Century-Crofts.

Weiss, C. (1984). Gender-related perceptions of caring in nurse–patient relationship. In M. Leininger (Ed.), *Care: The essence of nursing and health* (pp. 161–181). Thorofare, NJ: Charles B. Slack.

APPENDIX A: CARING BEHAVIOR CHECKLIST

Absent = 0
Present = 1

Verbal Caring Behaviors

Verbally responds to an expressed concern   ____

Explains procedure prior to initiation   ____

Verbally validates patient's physical status   ____

Verbally validates patient's emotional status   ____

Shares personal observations or feelings (self-disclosing) in response to patient's expression of concern   ____

Verbally reassures patient during care   ____

Discusses topics of patient's concern other than current health problem   ____

Nonverbal Caring Behaviors

Sits down at bedside   ____

Touches patient exclusive of procedure   ____

Sustains eye contact during patient interaction   ____

Enters patient's room without solicitation   ____

Provides physical comfort measures   ____

APPENDIX B: CLIENT PERCEPTION OF CARING SCALE

Directions: Please indicate how you feel by circling the number on a scale of 1 to 6

1. I felt that this nurse really listened to what I was saying.

1	2	3	4	5	6

Not at all   Very much

2. I felt reassured when this nurse cared for me.

1	2	3	4	5	6

Not at all   Very much

3. I felt that this nurse really valued me as an individual.

1	2	3	4	5	6

Not at all   Very much

4. I felt free to talk to this nurse about what concerned me.

1	2	3	4	5	6

Not at all   Very much

5. I felt the nurse was more interested in her "job" than my needs.

1	2	3	4	5	6

Not at all   Very much

6. I felt that this nurse could tell when something was bothering me.

1	2	3	4	5	6

Not at all   Very much

7. I felt secure with this nurse taking care of me.

1	2	3	4	5	6

Not at all   Very much

8. I felt frustrated by this nurse's attitude.

1	2	3	4	5	6

Not at all   Very much

9. I could tell this nurse really cared about me.

1	2	3	4	5	6

Not at all   Very much

10. I could tell that this nurse wanted to make me feel comfortable.

1	2	3	4	5	6

Not at all   Very much

18

Measuring Patient Satisfaction Outcomes Across Provider Disciplines

Gene W. Marsh

This chapter discusses the Patient Satisfaction with Health Care Provider Scale, a measure to compare patient satisfaction with health care providers from different disciplines working within the same primary care setting.

PURPOSE

Patient satisfaction ratings are subjective evaluations of health care providers and services that capture a personal evaluation of care that cannot be known by observing care directly (Ware, Snyder, Wright, & Davies, 1983). Although patient satisfaction instruments have proliferated in the past decade, noticeably absent from the literature is a reliable and valid tool for measuring patient satisfaction in primary care settings in which the health care providers' educational disciplines differ. Knowing how well patient expectations are met within alternative models that employ a mix of providers, such as HMOs, is critical for achieving high quality, cost-effective care. The Patient Satisfaction with Health Care Provider Scale (PSHCPS) was adapted and tested to measure and compare patient satisfaction with health care providers from different disciplines, such as nursing and medicine, working within the same primary care setting.

CONCEPTUAL BASIS: NURSING AND MEDICAL DIMENSIONS OF SATISFACTION

The concept of patient satisfaction frequently is included in studies of quality and cost outcomes. Patient satisfaction is fundamental to the quality of care because it provides information on the congruence between patients' expectations of providers and their perceptions of the actual care they receive (Donabedian, 1988). Others argue that patient satisfaction is more closely related to health service economics than to quality. Behaviors of dissatisfied individuals potentially affect both the individuals' quality of care outcomes as well as the provider and delivery system costs of providing care.

The nursing and medical literature were reviewed to determine if patient judgments of satisfaction with nursing and medical primary care providers share a similar conceptual foundation. Clarity of this conceptual point is critical for understanding if similar dimensions of satisfaction can adequately index the concept for both disciplines.

The most commonly measured dimensions of patient satisfaction in the medical literature are (1) physician's interpersonal manner and affect, including empathy and humaneness (caring), (2) physician's technical competence, (3) accessibility and convenience, and (4) finances or costs (Davies & Ware, 1991; DiMatteo & Hays, 1980; Fitzpatrick, 1991; Institute of Medicine (IOM), 1978; Kravitz, Cope, Bhrany, & Leake, 1994; Ross, Steward, & Sinacore, 1995; Safran, Tarlov, & Rogers, 1994; Stump, Dexter, Tierney, & Wolinsky, 1995; Ware, et al., 1983; Ware & Hays, 1988).

The transition of nurses from a physician-delegated to an independent or collaborative advanced practice role may underlie specification of dimensions that are currently similar to those associated with medicine. Technical competence, interpersonal competence, and caring dimensions are represented in the majority of nursing studies. Ability to share information, communicate knowledgeably and professionally, and involve patients and families in decision making about care are represented as both independent dimensions and dimensions that are imbedded in other primary care concepts. (Bond & Thomas, 1992; Forbes & Brown, 1995; La Monica, Oberst, Madea, & Wolf, 1986; Mansour & Al-Osimy, 1993; Petersen, 1988; Risser, 1975).

Risser's (1975) instrument, measuring patient satisfaction with primary care nurses in an outpatient setting, identifies four dimensions of patient satisfaction with primary care nurses: technical-professional competence, intrapersonal competence, trusting relationship, and educational relationship. Risser's research has influenced the development of other instruments measuring satisfaction in a variety of acute care and primary care settings (Giltinan & Murray, 1992; Hinshaw & Atwood, 1982; La Monica, et al., 1986).

Both nurse and medical researchers express concerns about the lack of conceptual independence between technical competence and interpersonal behaviors of nurses and physicians (DiMatteo & Hays, 1980; Donabedian, 1988; Health Services Research Group (HSRG), 1992; Petersen, 1988; Ware & Davies, 1983). Technical competence and interpersonal behaviors are moderately correlated ($r = .60$ to $.70$) (HSRG). Patients who are treated professionally and compassionately are more likely to overestimate technical competence (DiMatteo & Hays; Petersen; Ware & Hays, 1988).

Regardless of the provider's discipline, patients commonly evaluate how well care expectations are met on the following similar dimensions: technical competence, interpersonal competence (including caring affect, empathy, communication skills, ability to instill in the patient comfort, confidence, and trust in the provider), and ability to convey health care information. Accessibility, continuity of care, and cost are cited less frequently as dimensions of nursing care than of physician care.

PROCEDURE FOR ADAPTATION

The PSHCPS is adapted from the Patient Satisfaction Scale (PSS) developed by Cherkin, Hart, and Rosenblatt (1988). The PSS was originally derived from the Patient Satisfaction Questionnaire (PSQ) forms I and II (Ware, Davies-Avery, & Stewart, 1978; Ware, et al., 1983). The PSS is an 18-item scale comprising four subscales representing four dimensions of the PSQ (Ware, et al., 1983). The subscales measure General Satisfaction (four items, alpha = .84); Quality (six items, alpha = .69); Humaneness (six items alpha = .81); and Access (two items, alpha = .47). Cherkin et al. (1988) examined care perceptions of adult outpatients treated by family physicians (n = 213) and general internists (n = 218). They found no significant perceived differences in care based on the type of care provider.

In the adaptation, Marsh (1999) retained the item format, response options, and directionality of the PSS. However, for each item, the term "health care provider" replaces the term "doctor," and the term "health care" replaces "medical care" as indicated. Three new items were added to the Access subscale in an attempt to improve reliability. Marsh tested the 21-item PSHCPS among a sample of 167 indigent adult outpatients, randomly assigned to nurse practitioner and family practice physicians, at a large, university, managed care facility. Cronbach's alpha coefficients for the subscales were General Satisfaction .88; Quality .77; Humaneness .85; and Access .45.

Item Analysis and Reliability

Item analysis revealed that only three items exceeded interitem correlations of .70, suggesting that item redundancy was not inflating alpha. Three other items consistently failed to meet item-item (r = .30 to .70) and item-total (r > .40) criteria and were eliminated because they more closely measured system rather than provider characteristics. Interitem correlations ranged from .15 to .75 (M = .43). The total scale standardized Cronbach's alpha coefficient was .93.

Construct Validity

The 18-item revised PSHCPS was analyzed using factor analysis with a principal axis extraction and oblimin rotation (N = 167). Factor loading

TABLE 18.1 Factor Loadings for the Patient Satisfaction with Health Care Provider Scale (18 Items): Unrotated Principal Axis Factor Analysis

Item number	Factor loading
15	.84
14	.81
16	.77
6	.74
10	.70
12	.69
2	.68
17	.67
5	.62
4	.61
3	.61
13	.60
7	.60
8	.58
18	.54
9	.49
11	.46
1	.43

criteria were > .40 with a spread of .20 between factor loading scores with secondary factors. Exploratory findings revealed three factors with eigenvalues greater than 1 and explaining 59.3% of the total variance. However items from the expected underlying theoretical dimensions loaded across the three factors, and independent factors were not identified. A two-factor solution yielded similar results and provided evidence that the scale measured a single theoretical concept. A principal axis, unrotated solution, specifying one factor, confirmed that the data were best represented by a single factor. All factor loadings ranged from .43 to .84 with 43% of the variance explained (Table 18.1).

DESCRIPTION OF THE 18-ITEM PSHCPS

The 18-item revised Patient Satisfaction with Health Care Provider Scale is a unidimensional scale measuring a generalized conceptualization of patient satisfaction with primary care providers. Content, although originating from the medical discipline, also reflects patients' expectations of nursing care as reported in the nursing literature. The PSHCPS is a 5-point, summated rating scale. Response options are 1 = *strongly disagree*, 2 = *disagree*, 3 = *not sure*, 4 = *agree*, and 5 = *strongly agree*. Summated responses yield total scores with higher scores representing higher levels of satisfaction. The balanced number of positively and negatively worded items appears to minimize acquiescence response bias. However, the degree to which social desirability response bias exists is unknown (Marsh, 1999). The PSHCPS ranks at the 6.4 grade level on the Flesch-Kincaid Readability Test (Microsoft Word 97, 1997). The scale is self-administered and takes less than 10 minutes to complete.

ADMINISTRATION AND SCORING

The PSHCPS should be self-administered in a private location to minimize the risk of social response bias. Administering the PSHCPS as a mailed survey is not recommended when substantial time has elapsed between the health care encounter and point of measurement. Barton and Harrison (1998) received a 17.3% mailed response rate from 341 registered clients who sought care within the prior year at a nurse practitioner-run clinic. Additionally, instruments should be distributed and collected by a known, neutral, nonprovider. Consent procedures can be conducted while respondents are waiting for their appointments. Instruments should be completed immediately following the client/health provider encounter. Respondents are instructed to consider each item as a representation of the health care they have received from their health care provider even if they have seen the provider only once. Scores are assigned to items according to the scheme depicted in Table 18.2. The following eight items must be reverse coded: 4, 5, 7, 8, 12, 13, 16, and 17. A total score is achieved by summing across all items. Scores have a possible range of 18 to 90.

TABLE 18.2 PSHCPS Scoring Scheme for Positively Worded Items

Response	Symbol	Score
Strongly Agree	SA	5
Agree	A	4
Not Sure	NS	3
Disagree	D	2
Strongly Disagree	SD	1

RELIABILITY AND VALIDITY

Reliability

Internal consistency estimates of the PSHCPS across several studies range from Cronbach's alphas of .91 to .94. Reliability of the total scale is supported (Table 18.3).

Content Validity

Minor alterations of item wording and content have resulted in alternative forms of the PSHCPS that have yielded satisfactory results in various settings. Bezner, Canaday, and Davis (2000) modified the PSHCPS to evaluate client satisfaction in a nurse practitioner clinic serving primarily low-income children and young to middle-aged adults, 30% of whom were Spanish speaking only. Content validity was estimated by a panel of five experts according to procedures outlined by Lynn (1986). Fourteen items demonstrated content validity ranging from .80 to 1.00 and were retained with slight modifications. Four items were eliminated because they were not relevant to the sample and setting or did not meet content validity criteria. The term "health provider" was changed to "nurse practitioner." Because the response options seemed difficult for the popula tion, the options were changed to *yes, not sure,* and *no.* The 14 items were then translated and back translated by two bilingual professionals to develop a Spanish version. Both language versions were judged to be adequate for evaluating the outcome of nurse practitioner care.

Smith-Campbell (1996) studied the influence of a state funding policy on access to health care for the indigent in a Kansas county and used the PSHCPS as a subjective evaluation of the individual's experience with the health care system. She created a 7-item Access subscale by adding two additional items to Marsh's 21-item scale resulting in a 23-item revised scale. Findings revealed that the state policy influenced a reduction in the number of emergency department visits while satisfaction levels were moderately high (item $M = 4.2$.). Responses to the open-ended question, "Do you have additional comments about the services provided at this clinic?" were also positive and consistent with scale results.

Taylor (2000) revised the 18-item PSHCPS (Marsh, 1999) for use with patients receiving physical therapy (PT) by changing the term "health care provider" to "physiotherapist" and deleting items 9 and 11 as they were not relevant to PT. Taylor conducted a randomized controlled trial on patients receiving physical therapy for back pain in the United Kingdom. The PSHCPS was returned by 223 (75.6%) clients.

TABLE 18.3 Patient Satisfaction with Health Care Provider Scale: Evidence of Reliability and Validity

Study citation	Sample and characteristics	Reliability evidence	Validity evidence
Barton, A. & Harrison, A. (1998). *Nursing Clinic at Littleton, Advanced Training Grant, Annual Report,* USDHHS, Division of Nursing ID10 NU 30243–03.	*Sample size:* 51; 44.3% < 18 yrs; 23.3% 61–79 yrs. *Sample characteristics:* Nurse practitioner-run clinic with medically indigent target population.	*Internal consistency:* Total scale Cronbach's alpha = .92	
Bezner, S., Canaday, J., & Davis, N. (2000). *Evaluation of client satisfaction at the TWU CARES Clinic.* Unpublished Manuscript, Texas Women's University, Denton, TX.	*Sample size:* 35; males = 2, females = 28; unidentified = 5. *Sample characteristics:* M age = 51 yrs., S.D. = 13.5 yrs; English speaking = 27, Spanish speaking = 8. Nurse practitioner run clinic for low-income target population of children and young to mid-age adults.		*A priori content validity:* Using panel of 5 experts, 14/18 items met content validity criterion of ≥ .80 to 1.00. 14 items translated into Spanish and back translated.
Marsh, G. W. (1999). Measuring patient satisfaction outcomes across provider disciplines. *Journal of Nursing Measurement, 7* (1), 47–62.	*Sample size:* 167; males = 56, females = 104, unidentified = 7. *Sample characteristics:* Caucasian (127, 76%), African American (14, 8.4%), Hispanic (13, 7.8%), Asian (2, 1.2%), Other (3, 1.8%). Nurse	*Internal consistency:* Cronbach's alpha = .93 Interitem correlation range = .15–.75 (M = .42) Item to total correlation range = .41 to .83. Score M = 74.69, SD = 10.68	*A priori content validity:* 18 items generated from Cherkin et al., 1988; Ware et al., 1983. *Construct validity:* Confirmatory Factor analysis of one factor, 18 items, unrotated.

TABLE 18.3 *(continued)*

Study citation	Sample and characteristics	Reliability evidence	Validity evidence
Marsh (1999) *(continued)*	practitioner provider (92, 55.1%), Physician provider (66, 39.5%); urban managed care setting for the medically indigent.	Subscale Cronbach's alphas for 21-item scale: General Satisfaction = .88 Quality = .77 Humaneness = .85 Access = .45 *Response Bias:* Positive and negative item responses in expected directions.	Factor loading scores range = .43 to .84. No sig. differences between provider types ($F = .58$; $df = 1, 145$; $p = .45$) expected result.
Smith-Campbell, B. (1996). *Access: Effects of a state funded policy in one community.* Unpublished doctoral dissertation, University of Colorado, Health Sciences Center, Denver.	*Sample size:* 153; males = 35; females = 118. *Sample characteristics:* Caucasian (124, 81%), African Am. (14, 9.2%) Hispanic (12, 8.2%), Native Am. (1, .7%), Other (14, 9.2%). Age 18–34 (50%), 35–44 (26%), 45+ (24%). Education: some H. S. or less (22.89%), H. S. grad to some college (58.6%), College grad. (18.5%). Income: < $9,999 (66.9%), $10,000—$19,999 (30.5%), $20,000—$39,999 (2.6%).	*Internal consistency:* Total scale (23-items) Cronbach's alpha = .91 *Subscale* Cronbach's alphas for 23-item scale: General Satisfaction = .88 Quality = .78 Humaneness = .85 Access = .67	*Content validity:* Smith-Campbell (1996) retained the original subscale structure (Marsh, 1999) and added 2 items to the access subscale. Congruence between item responses and open ended qualitative responses

TABLE 18.3 (*continued*)

Study citation	Sample and characteristics	Reliability evidence	Validity evidence
	Nurse practitioner provider (74.7%), physician provider (13.3%), physician assistant provider (8.2%), RN provider (3.8%). Target population, state funded primary care services for the medically indigent.		
Taylor, S. (2000). *Does provision of telephone advice improve patient satisfaction with a physiotherapy service?* Unpublished Master of Science thesis, University of Northumbria, Newcastle, UK.	*Sample size:* 223; males = 77, females = 146. *Sample characteristics:* age 14—91 yrs. Patients of two large National Health Service general practices in urban Northeastern England with back pain, referred for physical therapy tx. Experimental intervention group ($n = 99$); Control group ($n = 124$)	*Internal consistency:* Total scale Cronbach's alpha = .94	*Content validity:* Deleted items 9 and 11 as not relevant for physical therapy practice. *Construct validity:* Hypothesis that experimental group would be significantly more satisfied with physical therapy services supported by Mann Whitney U analysis ($p = .000$)

Construct Validity

Although evidence supported reliability of three of the four PSHCPS subscales, factor analysis failed to demonstrate the existence of more than one factor. Preliminary analyses revealed correlations among the General Satisfaction, Quality, and Humaneness subscales ranging from .70 to .77. The high degree of correlation might indicate that the three factors measure a single theoretical concept (Marsh, 1999). Based on confirmatory factor analysis results with deletion of three weak items, Marsh determined that the PSHCPS is a unidimensional scale and recommends using the 18-item revised scale as presented in the Appendix to this chapter.

Discriminability

In one study, Marsh (1999) used the PSHCPS as intended to compare perceived satisfaction across different types of providers. The finding that there were no perceived differences in satisfaction by provider type was expected ($F = .58$; df 1,145; $p = .45$).

To determine if the PSHCPS would discriminate between those highest and lowest in satisfaction, Marsh (1999) conducted a t-test comparing mean satisfaction levels for the lowest and highest quartiles of the distribution. The results of the independent t test revealed no statistically significant difference in patient satisfaction between the least and most satisfied individuals of the distribution ($t = -.70$, $p = .49$).

In contrast, ability of the PSHCPS to discriminate between lower and higher levels of satisfaction was evident in a study by Taylor (2000). In this study, patients from two large general practices in urban Northeast England ($N = 295$) were referred by their general practitioners to PT for the treatment of back pain and were randomly assigned to an experimental or control group. During the interim between the referral and encounter with the physical therapist, the experimental group received a telephone intervention from a physical therapist on self-management of back pain. Analysis using the Mann-Whitney U statistical test supported the hypothesis that the experimental group would be significantly more satisfied with physical therapy services ($p = .000$).

CONCLUSIONS AND RECOMMENDATIONS

Evidence from research assessing the 18-item Patient Satisfaction with Health Care Provider Scale provides support for its reliability and validity as a unidimensional scale with item content indexing satisfaction with provider characteristics. Smith-Campbell (1996) also found the scale suitable for measuring satisfaction at the system level.

Factor analysis results support a unidimensional scale structure. Several researchers (Donabedian, 1988; Risser, 1975; Ware et al., 1983) posit that patient satisfaction should be conceptualized as a multidimensional construct. According to Ware et al. (1983), if there are distinct features of health care services that cause differences in patient satisfaction, such as cost and access, then a valid measure of satisfaction needs to be multidimensional. Marsh's (1999) conceptualization of patient satisfaction was focused narrowly, primarily, and intentionally on provider characteristics, and underrepresents the full patient satisfaction content domain reflected in the literature. The narrow provider focus of satisfaction in Marsh's research, indistinct theoretical boundaries between provider technical and interpersonal competence described in the literature, and limited subscale discrimination in previous research create plausible explanations for the failure to identify multiple dimensions in the PSHCPS.

Because patient satisfaction is viewed as an indicator of quality and an indirect indicator of cost, the PSHCPS may potentially be suitable for measurement from either perspective. The conceptual perspective of patient satisfaction as either a quality or economic indicator will dictate whether the concept should be studied as a dependent or independent variable (Donabedian, 1988; Ware & Davies, 1983). Studied as a dependent variable, patient satisfaction ratings contain useful information about the structure, process, and outcomes of care. Studying satisfaction as an independent variable may be useful in predicting patient care-seeking, adherence, and reactive behaviors, including those behaviors that have a negative impact on health provider and system costs (Ware & Davies, 1983). The PSHCPS also potentially may be valuable in health services and clinical outcomes research when it is useful to evaluate patient satisfaction outcomes with alternative models of care delivery that employ providers from different disciplines.

Continuing research is warranted to address the following issues: (1) clarity around the PSHCPS's ability to discriminate between satisfied and dissatisfied clients; (2) sensitivity of the PSHCPS in detecting changes in satisfaction over time; and (3) suitability for use by disciplines other than nursing, medicine, or physical therapy. Additional item revision may enhance the scale's relevancy for other disciplines. For example, item 11 could be replaced with a more relevant index of lifestyle across disciplines such as, "my health care provider advises me about my lifestyle practices."

Initial instrument testing and research with the PSHCPS demonstrate that it is a useful indicator of patient satisfaction with nurse and physician primary care providers working collaboratively or within the same setting and also within a physical therapy setting. System variables such as access, cost, and convenience may be better assessed with alternative, conceptually broader instruments. The scale also appears suitable for use in evaluating outcomes of nurse practitioner care and other unique provider types when comparisons between provider types are indicated. The PSH-

CPS has demonstrated suitability for use with low-income, medically indigent clients and client groups with varying socioeconomic levels as well as English- and Spanish-speaking Americans and British clients. Scale results should continue to be interpreted cautiously as future study is warranted to address continuing reliability and validity issues.

REFERENCES

Barton, A., & Harrison, A. (1998). *Nursing clinic at Littleton, advanced training grant, annual report,* (U. S. Department of Health and Human Services, Division of Nursing ID10 NU 30243–03). Washington, DC: USDHHS.

Bezner, S., Canaday, J., & Davis, N. (2000). *Evaluation of client satisfaction at the TWU CARES Clinic.* Unpublished Manuscript, Texas Woman's University, Denton, TX.

Bond, S., & Thomas, L. H. (1992). Measuring patients' satisfaction with nursing care. *Journal of Advanced Nursing, 17,* 52–63.

Cherkin, D. C., Hart, L. G., & Rosenblatt, R. A. (1988). Patient satisfaction with family physicians and general internists: Is there a difference? *The Journal of Family Practice, 26 ,* 543–551.

Davies, A. R., & Ware, J. E. (1991). *GHAA's consumer satisfaction survey and user's manual.* Washington DC: Group Health Association of America

DiMatteo, M. R., & Hays, R. (1980). The significance of patients' perceptions of physician conduct: A study of patient satisfaction in a family practice center. *Journal of Community Health, 6,* 18–34.

Donabedian, A. (1988). The quality of care: How can it be assessed? *Journal of the American Medical Association, 260,* 1743–1748.

Fitzpatrick, R. (1991). Surveys of patient satisfaction: I—Important general considerations. *British Medical Journal, 302,* 887–889.

Forbes, M. L., & Brown, H. N. (1995). Developing an instrument for measuring patient satisfaction. *Association of Perioperative Registered Nurses, 61,* 737–743.

Giltinan, J. M., & Murray, K. T. (1992). Meeting the health care needs of the rural elderly: Client satisfaction with a university-sponsored nursing center. *Journal of Rural Health, 8,* 305–310.

Health Services Research Group (HSRG) (1992). A guide to direct measures of patient satisfaction in clinical practice. *Canadian Medical Association Journal, 146,* 1727–1731.

Hinshaw, A. S., & Atwood, J. R. (1982). A patient satisfaction instrument: Precision by replication, *Nursing Research, 31,* 170–175.

Institute of Medicine (IOM) (1978). *Report of a study: A manpower policy for primary health care.* Washington DC: National Academy of Sciences.

Kravitz, R. L., Cope, D. W., Bhrany, V., & Leake, B. (1994). Internal medicine patients' expectations for care during office visits. *Journal of General Internal Medicine, 9,* 75–81.

La Monica, E. L., Oberst, M. T., Madea, A. R., & Wolf, R. M. (1986). Development of a patient satisfaction scale. *Research in Nursing & Health, 9,* 43–50.

Lynn, M. (1986). Determination and quantification of content validity. *Nursing Research, 35,* 382–385.

Mansour, A. A., & Al-Osimy, M. H. (1993). A study of satisfaction among primary health care patients in Saudi Arabia. *Journal of Community Health, 18,* 163–173.

Marsh, G. W. (1999). Measuring patient satisfaction outcomes across provider disciplines. *Journal of Nursing Measurement, 7(1),* 47–62.

Microsoft Word 97 (Computer software) (1997). Seattle: Microsoft Corporation.

Petersen, M. B. H. (1988). Measuring patient satisfaction: Collecting useful data. *Journal of Nursing Quality Assurance, 2(3),* 25–35.

Risser, N. (1975). Development of an instrument to measure patient satisfaction with nurses and nursing care in primary care settings. *Nursing Research, 24,* 45–52.

Ross, C. K., Steward, C. A., & Sinacore, J. M. (1995). A comparative study of seven measures of patient satisfaction. *Medical Care, 33,* 392–406.

Safran, D. G., Tarlov, A. R., & Rogers, W. H. (1994). Primary care performance in fee-for-service and prepaid health care systems: Results from the Medical Outcomes Study. *Journal of the American Medical Association, 271,* 1579–1586.

Smith-Campbell, B. (1996). *Access: Effects of a state funded policy in one community.* Unpublished doctoral dissertation, University of Colorado, Health Sciences Center, Denver.

Stump, T. E., Dexter, P. R., Tierney, W. M., & Wolinsky, F. D. (1995). Measuring patient satisfaction with physicians among older and diseased adults in a primary care municipal outpatient setting: An examination of three instruments. *Medical Care, 33,* 958–972.

Taylor, S. (2000). *Does provision of telephone advice improve patient satisfaction with a physiotherapy service?* Unpublished Master of Science thesis, University of Northumbria, Newcastle, UK.

Ware, J. E., & Davies, A. R. (1983). Behavioral consequences of consumer dissatisfaction with medical care. *Evaluation and Program Planning, 6,* 291–297.

Ware, J. E., Davies-Avery, A., & Stewart, A. L. (1978). The measurement and meaning of patient satisfaction. *Health and Medical Care Services Review, 1(1),* 3–15.

Ware, J. E., & Hays, R. D. (1988). Methods for measuring patient satisfaction with specific medical encounters. *Medical Care, 26,* 393–402.

Ware, J. E., Snyder, M. K., Wright, W. R., & Davies, A. R. (1983). Defining and measuring patient satisfaction with medical care. *Evaluation and Program Planning 6,* 247–2634

APPENDIX: PATIENT SATISFACTION WITH
HEALTH CARE PROVIDER SCALE

INSTRUCTIONS: Following are some statements about your health care. Please read each one carefully, keeping in mind the care you have received from your health care provider, even if you have seen him or her only once. Circle the letters to the right of each question that best indicates how you feel about your ability to get the health care you need.

Strongly Agree	= SA
Agree	= A
Not Sure	= NS
Disagree	= D
Strongly Disagree	= SD

Item	Rating
1. If I have a health care question, I can reach my health care provider for help without any problem.	SA A NS D SD
2. My health care provider always does his or her best to keep me from worrying.	SA A NS D SD
3. My health care provider always treats me with respect.	SA A NS D SD
4. Sometimes my health care provider makes me feel foolish.	SA A NS D SD
5. My health care provider causes me to worry a lot because he or she doesn't explain medical problems to me.	SA A NS D SD
6. My health care provider respects my feelings.	SA A NS D SD
7. My health care provider hardly ever explains my medical problems to me.	SA A NS D SD
8. My health care provider is not as thorough as he or she should be.	SA A NS D SD
9. My health care provider encourages me to get a yearly exam.	SA A NS D SD
10. My health care provider is very careful to check everything when examining me.	SA A NS D SD
11. My health care provider asks what foods I eat and explains why certain foods are best.	SA A NS D SD
12. My health care provider ignores medical problems I've had in the past when I seek care for new problems.	SA A NS D SD
13. My health care provider doesn't explain about ways to avoid illness or injury.	SA A NS D SD

14. I'm very satisfied with the care I receive from
    my health care provider.   SA A NS D SD
15. The care I receive from my health care
    provider is just about perfect.   SA A NS D SD
16. My health care provider could give better care.   SA A NS D SD
17. There are things about the care I receive from
    my health care provider which could be better. SA A NS D SD
18. The type of health care I need is available
    from my health care provider.   SA A NS D SD

For permission to use or revise this scale contact: Gene W. Marsh RN, PhD, Associate Professor, University of Colorado Health Sciences Center, School of Nursing, C-288, 4200 East Ninth Avenue, Denver, Colorado 80262 (303) 315–1164. e-mail gene.marsh@uchsc.edu

Citation: Marsh, G. W. (1999). Measuring patient satisfaction outcomes across provider disciplines. *Journal of Nursing Management* 7(1), 47–62.

19

Measuring Outcomes of Home Health Care: The Episode Coding Form

Janet I. Feldman and Robert J. Richard

This chapter discusses an Episode Coding Form for evaluating nursing outcomes in home health care agencies.

PURPOSE

Although the discipline of nursing has at least a 30–year history of research devoted to problems, issues, and concern with the allocation of nursing services, there are still questions of quality, productivity, and care outcomes. The goal of this work, part of a larger study of home health care, was to develop quantitative measures of the nursing care status of elderly patients at the beginning and again at the end of episodes of home care. The result is a patient classification method based on nursing diagnosis-like statements. An overall classification score reflects both the number of nursing problems/diagnoses unresolved at the end of an episode of care and the difficulty of remaining at home with such problems. It summarizes scores in four major problem areas, which in turn include a total of 22 subscale scores.

CONCEPTUAL BASIS

A definition of patient/nursing care outcomes may be found in *Health Care at Home: An Essential Component of a National Health Policy* (American Nurses Association, 1978): "Outcomes are measures of alteration in health status. For the patient, an outcome criterion would be a measurable change in the state of his/her health. Outcomes may be positive or negative and are the ultimate indicators of quality care" (p. 13). According to Rowland and Rowland (1980) such criteria for health care outcomes have been fairly well agreed on and thus are attractive because of face validity. The first step in the development of the classification score for an outcome measure was a computerized literature search.

Only two reports of classification systems were found that assessed patients for home health care. The first was a method used by Daubert (1979) in a nursing outcome study. The second classified the patient's functional status for the purpose of determining the need for nursing resources (Fortinsky, Granger, & Seltzer, 1981).

Giovannetti (1978) stated that there were no patient classification systems in general use in community health nursing as late as 1978. Simmons (1980) developed a classification scheme that provided a uniform nomenclature for identifying client problems in community nursing. The statements used by Simmons closely resembled those used by Daubert (1979). They were obvious precursors for what since has become nursing diagnostic statements (Gordon, 1982). Indeed, Simmons stated that her problem statements resembled nursing diagnoses and that work was ongoing to transform this scheme into a method for assessing nursing outcomes. The Simmons format and conceptual framework were chosen for this study to measure nursing care outcomes. Simmons describes this classification scheme as

> an orderly arrangement of a nonexhaustive list of patient problems diagnosed by nurses in a community health setting . . . subdivided into four major domains each including the names of problems identified in each domain . . . modifiers of the problems and signs and symptoms of the problems . . . The four major domains of classification scheme represent broad areas of patient problems which are addressed by the community health nurse. The four domains are environmental, psycho-social, physiological and health behaviors. The patient problems are grouped within these four major domains. Problems are described by a cluster of signs and symptoms which are listed beneath each problem in the scheme. The signs or symptoms are general statements which condense more specific information about the patient. (p. 6)

These considerations provided a specific rationale for using this particular scheme. It was used (with several modifications) to develop a rudimentary patient classification method for home health patients aged 65 and older.

PROCEDURES FOR DEVELOPMENT

Data were obtained from closed patient care records of 12 home care agencies in one midwestern state. The agencies represented one each of four ownership groups (not-for-profit, proprietary, hospital-based, and health department) in three locations (rural, suburban, and small city). The 436 cases reviewed were a 10% random sample of the unduplicated censuses of the 12 agencies. Patients under age 65 were excluded. The data included the standard demographic information for the patients as well as items describing the independency level and problems and needs at the beginning and end of each episode of care during the study year. There were a total of 528 care episodes for the 436 patients.

An edited version of the Simmons (1980) problem list was used to abstract and then code each patient's status and situation at the beginning and end of each episode of care. Three adjustments were made to adapt and edit the problem list for the coding. First, those items that did not pertain to patients over age 65 were deleted. This reduced the problem/ nursing diagnoses list to 199 items. Second, this list was given to a panel of three experts who weighted them by making a judgment on each individual item in relation to the question, How serious is this problem for an older individual in relation to his/her ability to function at home? The weights that the panel was asked to use were: 1 = *not very serious*, 2 = *moderately serious*; and 3 = *very serious*.

The three nursing experts who assisted in this included two Ph.D.-prepared nurses and a master's-prepared nurse clinical specialist in gerontological nursing. One of the doctorally prepared nurses had extensive background in anatomy and has done clinical work and teaching in gerontological nursing and research in gerontological microanatomy. The master's-prepared nurse has worked with gerontological patients for the past five years and was currently an instructor of gerontological nursing in a university setting.

An analysis was done to ascertain how often the three panel members agreed or disagreed on the weights for individual items. The results were that the three nurses assigned the same weight to 58 items (29%). For 126 items (63%), two of three nurses assigned the same weight, and 15 items (8%) were weighted differently by the three nurses. Overall for 184 of the 199 items (92%), two out of the three nurses or all three nurses agreed as to the weight to be assigned to the items. This high level of agreement as to the weight, or seriousness, of the particular problem/ nursing diagnosis of an elderly individual's functional status at home provided some additional assurance that the items did in fact reflect the problems and/or needs of a home health patient and that the problem classification scheme could be used with the weights as a patient classification method suitable for the purposes of the larger study. These assigned weights were averaged for each of the items.

Unfortunately, 199 statements were still too many for data analysis. The weighted statements were reviewed two more times with additional criteria in mind: (1) how frequently, in the opinion of the researchers, had this statement appeared during data collection; (2) what subtlety of information would be lost if a statement were combined or subsumed into a higher level descriptor; (3) would it really matter if the more detailed descriptor was subsumed; and (4) was it urgent that this particular level of detail be represented in this study or that this particular need/problem be at a fine level of detail. The result was a final total of 111 items. These items were assigned either the original weights or, when the statements were subsumed or adapted into more general descriptors, the average weights. A single data collector was used.

ADMINISTRATION AND SCORING

These adaptations of the original Simmons problem list were pilot tested. The total average time to abstract a single home care record was less than 20 minutes, while the time to abstract a single episode of care (start and end) averaged about 10 minutes. The admission visit and two subsequent visits were abstracted for the start classification data, and the last or discharge visit and two prior visits were used for the end classification data. Each episode of care was coded separately. If a patient had had one episode of care during the fiscal year, then one such coding form was completed. If the patient had had five episodes of care during the fiscal year, then five episode forms were completed. The 111 need/problem statements were answered either yes (1) or no (0).

The category of "unknown" was subsumed into the no answer, or 0. This coding decision masked an important issue for this retrospective record review: whether or not the original records might be a reliable and valid picture of the patient and the health care provided. Usually, the category "unknown" has meant that there was no possible way to find this particular information at the agency. In this instance, due to the coding decision, it was categorized as no. In other words, a presumption was made that if the problem was not noted, charted, or indicated in some way, it in fact did not exist. As there was no way to check such an existence, it was perceived as the only reasonable position. In contrast to "unknown," missing data (code 8) represented the data collector's own field coding and data collection errors. Thus, where 8 had to be coded, it was in no way a reflection on the agency's records.

In addition, a format to assess the agency records was devised as a method to alleviate a concern about the adequacy of the records used as a data source. The form was filled out at the completion of the data collection period in the agency. In essence, the form listed those factors, components, and issues that a basic nursing text (Wolff, Weitzel, & Fuerst, 1979) indicated as fundamental to adequate, appropriate, and legally correct charting in any health care agency. A general ranking of the agencies in relation to the adequacy, convenience, and correctness of their records, as assessed by a nonemployee health professional, indicated that three could be categorized as superior, six very good, and three fair. None of the original sample agencies had to be replaced because of poor records.

The next step was the formation of a linear scale by summing the weighted responses. First, each item as coded (0 = no; 1 = yes) was multiplied by the assigned weight to obtain the item value. Second, all of the item values for each of the subscales were summed to obtain the subscale values. Third, all subscale totals were summed for each major scale value. Finally, the major scale values were summed to produce the classification score for either the beginning or the end of a case episode.

The goal was the development of an overall patient classification index that would be applicable at both the beginning and the end of a care episode. The 111 items were organized into a hierarchy of subscales using the framework from the Simmons (1980) study. The resulting four scales for the classification index reflected the original conceptual framework: environment, psychosocial, physiological, and health behaviors. Table 19.1 includes the item assignments and weights for the index. The Episode Code Form can be found in the Appendix.

RELIABILITY AND VALIDITY

This overall index (PTCLASS) required several steps, as intermediate subscales were formed due to the large number of items involved. The final PTCLASS index was made up of the four scales. These were devised by combining 22 subscales based on the original 111 items. One of the major scales, Environment, did not require the formation of subscales as there were only a few items. Using the Statistical Package for the Social Science (SPSS) (Nie, Hull, Jenkins, Steinbrenner, & Bent, 1970) programs, Pearson's correlations were obtained for each of the initial 22 subscales and the four major scales. The correlations were reviewed, and where the researchers felt that some improvement in the r could be obtained, items were reassigned. No items were dropped from the subscales.

Lower correlations were found when there were scales that included items that were conceptually related from a nursing point of view but whose origin reflected different disciplines. This was not unanticipated, as a number of authors and researchers reporting on the development of patient classification systems described this and similar problems (Chagon, Audette, Lebrun, & Tilquin, 1978; Connor, 1964; Des Ormeaux, 1977; Leatt, Kyung, & Stinson, 1981; McPhail, 1975; Overton, Harrison, & Stinson, 1977; Parker & Boyd, 1974; Plummer, 1976; Roehrl, 1979; Tilquin, 1976; Trivedi, 1979). In general, the subscales with a strong biophysical orientation had higher inter-item correlations than those concerned with psychosocial factors.

Then the PTCLASS index was tested for reliability. For this correlational analysis, the data of 528 episodes of care from all 12 agencies were used. This was done because the original frequency distributions for each

TABLE 19.1 Subscale Item Assignment and Weights for Patient
Classification Scale

Scale	Weight
Environment	
Income deficit	2.33
Sanitation deficit	2.25
Residence safety hazard	2.06
Psychosocial	
Subscale: Maladaptive Behaviors, Grief	
Language barrier/dissatisfied with services	1.33
Social isolation	1.58
Suspicious behavior pattern	1.66
Compulsive behavior pattern	1.33
Role change	1.11
Interpersonal conflict	1.83
Grief	1.40
Subscale: Confusion	
Confusion: attention span	1.60
Confusion: time, place, person	2.33
Confusion: forgetfulness	1.33
Subscale: Depression	
Feeling of hopelessness/worthlessness	2.00
Excessive inward focus	2.00
Expresses wish to die	1.66
Fails to meet personal needs	2.00
Subscale: Anxiety, caretaking	
Feeling of apprehension	1.66
Irritable	1.33
Much purposeless activity	1.33
Lacks caretaking skills	2.66
Lacks consistent routine for caretaking	2.00
Neglect	1.90
Abuse	2.05
Behavior inappropriate for age	1.33
Physiological	
Subscale: Sensory, Communication	
Hearing impairment	1.41
Vision impairment	1.52
Lacks ability to speak	2.00
Inability to understand	2.66
Relies on nonverbal communication	2.00
Dentition impairment	2.00

TABLE 19.1 *(continued)*

Scale	Weight
Subscale: Respiratory	
Abnormal breath patterns (SOB/dyspnea)	1.66
Cough	1.00
Cyanosis	2.33
Noisy respiration	2.00
Rhinorrhea	1.00
Abnormal breath sounds	2.00
Subscale: Circulatory	
Edema	2.00
Cramping/pain in extremities	2.00
Decreased pulses	2.66
Discoloration of skin/cyanosis	2.33
Temperature change in affected areas	2.00
Varicosities	1.00
Fainting/syncopal episodes	3.00
Abnormal blood pressure	1.66
Pulse deficit	2.00
Irregular heart rate	1.66
Excessive rapid/slow heart rate	2.00
Reports anginal pain	3.00
Abnormal heart sounds	1.66
Subscale: Mobility, musculoskeletal	
Limited ROM/contractures	1.33
Poor coordination	2.00
Gait/ambulation disturbance	2.00
Decreased muscle strength/muscle tightness	1.66
Inability to manage ADL	3.00
Tremors	2.00
Subscale: Gastrointestinal	
Nausea/vomiting	3.00
Difficulty chewing/swallowing	2.33
Indigestion/heartburn	1.66
Anorexia	2.33
Anemia	2.00
Abnormal weight loss	2.66
Subscale: Lifestyle	
Inability to cope with body changes	1.83
Lifestyle incongruent with physiological changes	1.83
Subscale: Bowel	
Diarrhea	2.66
Constipation	1.66
Pain with defecation	1.66

TABLE 19.1 *(continued)*

Scale	Weight
Subscale: Bowel *(continued)*	
Minimal bowel sounds	1.66
Blood in stool	2.66
Abnormal colon	2.33
Cramping/abdominal discomfort	2.00
Increased frequency of stools	1.66
Incontinent of stools	2.66
Subscale: Bladder	
Incontinent of urine	2.66
Urgency/frequency	2.00
Burning/painful urination	1.66
Inability to empty bladder	2.33
Nocturia	1.66
Polyuria	2.00
Oliguria	2.00
Hematuria	2.66
Subscale: Skin	
Lesion (wound/burn/incision)	2.00
Rash	1.66
Inflammation	2.00
Drainage	2.33
Subscale: Pain	
Pain: client statement	2.33
Pain: elevated pulse, respiration, BP	2.33
Pain: compensatory movement	2.33
Pain: pallor, sweating	2.66
Lacks response to normal stimuli	3.00
Health Behaviors	
Subscale: Nutrition	
Abnormal intake of essential food/fluids	2.00
Emaciated/obese	2.33
Subscale: Sleep	
Awakens frequently	1.00
Insufficient rest/sleep	2.33
Subscale: Lifestyle/Personal Hygiene	
Sedentary life-style	1.33
'Inappropriate exercise	2.00
Personal hygiene deficit	1.44
Substance misuses	2.83
Subscale: Compliance, Knowledge, Weight Skill	
Noncompliance with medical visits	1.58
Noncompliance with Rx	1.66

TABLE 19.1 *(continued)*

Scale	Weight
Fails to obtain necessary equipment	1.66
Deviates from prescribed dosage	2.33
Lacks system for taking medication	2.00
Medications improperly stored	3.00
Does not obtain med refills	2.00
Unable to integrate diet into balanced nutrition	2.00
Does not adhere to diet Rx	1.66
Unable to demonstrate/relate procedure accurately	2.00
Requires nursing skill	2.33
Unable to perform procedure without assistance	2.66
Unable to operate special equipment properly	2.66

of the 111 items indicated that with a few "exceptions," the yes responses were under 25% per item. Thus it seemed unlikely that any one or even two of the agencies would provide enough responses for analysis. The goals were to build a single scale with internal consistency appropriate to the hierarchical framework used and to identify, insofar as time and money permitted, multiple item indicators for each subscale of each subdomain.

Since neither stability nor equivalence was a design issue, the coefficient alpha (Cronbach's alpha) was the method used to determine reliability. To accomplish this, the various subscale totals were used as the variables to test the reliability of the major scales. Table 19.2 presents these reliability coefficients. It is to be noted that the reliability coefficients reported represent major scales created from subscales used as items versus the alternative of major scales made from the individual 111 items.

The reliability coefficient of the PTCLASS index was a Cronbach's alpha of .48. Again, this index was created from the four major scale

TABLE 19.2 Reliability Coefficients (Cronbach's alpha) for Start and End Major Scales

Major scale	alpha (start)	alpha (end)
Environment	.56	.70
Psychosocial	.46	.63
Physiological	.39	.65
Health Behaviors	.24	.40

totals rather than the individual items. The interpretation was that the index was moderately reliable, as alpha values of .70 to .89 or higher are indicative of reliable scales. Face validity of the index was assumed, as it was conceptually based on previous works where this issue had been addressed and tested (Simmons, 1980).

Next, separate PTCLASS scales were defined for each episode of care at two points in time. The Start Patient Classification, SPTCLASS, used the data that described patient care/nursing needs at the beginning of an episode of care, and the End Patient Classification, EPTCLASS, used identically weighted items to describe the patient care nursing needs and problems unresolved and/or identifiable at the end of each episode of home care. These two scales were also tested for reliability: EPTCLASS obtained a Cronbach's alpha of .55, and SPTCLASS an alpha of .48. The two linear scales, SPTCLASS and EPTCLASS, were then used to assess the aggregated episode data of each of the 12 home health agencies.

Mean SPTCLASS and EPTCLASS scores were defined for each home health agency. These mean scores represented the average nursing care problems and/or nursing diagnoses and needs at the beginning and end of an episode of care for the subject-patients of each agency. A high numerical score indicated many nursing problems and therefore a high need for nursing care. Paired t-tests were used to compare the start and the classification mean scores for each agency.

The null hypothesis was that no difference between the start classification score and the end classification score for each of the 12 agencies would be found. The results of the paired t-tests were that the null hypothesis had to be rejected 11 out of 12 times (p = .05). These results indicated that there were statistically significant differences between start and end classification scores for all but one agency. This agency had an end classification mean score that was higher than the start classification mean score. This was an agency that had a high recidivism rate to the hospital. Table 19.3 presents the sample size, mean, and standard deviation for the two classification mean scores and *t*-values of the 12 agencies.

CONCLUSION AND RECOMMENDATIONS

The conclusions reached regarding this method for measuring nursing care outcomes were the following:

1. The patient classification methods themselves were moderately reliable. The end classification score was more reliable than the start classification score.
2. The reliability for the subscales was not as high as it might have been. The psychosocial items included in several of the subscales caused problems and difficulties in achieving good internal consis-

TABLE 19.3 Paired *t*-tests for Agency Start and End Classification Mean Scores

Agency	N	M (start)	SD (start)	M (end)	SD (end)	t
1	61	25.86	13.03	17.23	16.97	4.56*
2	22	7.20	4.16	4.39	5.89	3.16*
3	37	15.04	11.42	15.46	14.97	-.30
4	77	19.43	12.62	12.03	13.49	4.42*
5	115	16.22	9.52	9.71	13.93	6.39*
6	40	16.79	6.67	8.03	7.92	5.71*
7	16	22.10	12.28	3.79	6.89	5.30*
8	61	14.83	6.83	5.65	8.78	7.84*
9	64	22.52	12.79	11.79	14.78	7.21*
10	10	20.29	5.15	5.81	5.47	6.70*
11	10	20.36	7.27	7.11	6.83	4.35*
12	15	23.10	11.39	7.088	10.21	4.39*

*$p = .05$.

tency. The psychosocial items fit the scales in terms of nursing concepts but did not foster statistical reliability. The problem with psychosocial items was not unusual, as it had been noted by Connor (1964) when the first patient classification systems were developed.
3. The trend for 11 of the 12 agencies was that the end classification mean scores were lower than the start classification mean scores for this sample. This was interpreted to mean that the subjects had on average fewer nursing care problems at the end of an episode of home care than at the beginning.
4. Using these measures, a statistical difference was demonstrable between the beginning and end of an episode of home care for elderly patients.
5. The end classification mean scores could be considered as an indicator of care outcomes for home care at an agency level.
6. Additional refinements were needed for the subscales and for the start and end indices, including additional revisions and field testing.

These refinements should include using fewer items to achieve the same or improved reliability coefficients, or, at minimum, another review of the present correlation coefficients. Revision of the subscales might include the reassignment of items, the addition and/or deletion of items to update the indices to reflect the current changes in home health care practice, and the prospective testing of the patient classification at one or more of the other home care classification systems now emerging. A future field test could also include using the scales on an individual patient basis to assess care outcomes rather than in the aggregate, as was done in this study.

REFERENCES

American Nurses' Association (1978). *Health care at home: An essential component of a national health policy.* Kansas City, MO: Author.

Chagon, M., Audette, L. M., Lebrun, L., & Tilquin, C. (1978). A patient classification system by level of nursing care required. *Nursing Research, 27*, 103–113.

Connor, R. H. (1964). Hospital inpatient classification system. *Dissertation Abstracts International, 183364.* (University Microfilms No. 60–3319).

Daubert, E. A. (1979). Patient classification system and outcome criteria. *Nursing Outlook, 27*, 450–454.

Des Ormeaux, S. P. (1977). Implementation of the C.A.S.H. patient classification system for staffing determination. *Supervisor Nurse, 8*(4), 29–35.

Feldman, J., & Richard, R. J. (1988). A measure of nursing outcomes for home health care. In C. F. Waltz & O. L. Strickland (Eds.), *Measurement of nursing outcomes: Vol. 1: Measuring client outcomes* (pp. 475–495). New York: Springer Publishing Co.

Fortinsky, R. H., Granger, C. V., & Seltzer, G. B. (1981). The use of functional assessment in understanding home care needs. *Medical Care, 19,* 489–497.

Giovannetti, P. (1978). *Patient classification systems in nursing: A description and analysis* (DHEW Publication No. HRA 78022). Washington DC: U.S. Government Printing Office.

Gordon, M. (1982). *Manual of nursing diagnosis.* New York: McGraw-Hill.

Leatt, P., Kyung, S. B., & Stinson, S. M. (1981). An instrument for assessing and classifying patients by types of care. *Nursing Research, 30*, 145–150.

McPhail, A. (1975). The meaning of patient classification. *Dimensions in Health Services, 52*(6), 30–39.

Nie, N. H., Hull, C. H., Jenkins, J. G., Steinbrenner, K., & Bent, D. H. (1970). *Statistical package for the social sciences* (2nd ed.). New York: McGraw-Hill.

Overton, P., Harrison, F., & Stinson, S. (1977). Patient classification by types of care. *Dimensions in Health Services, 54*(8), 27–30.

Parker, R., & Boyd, J. (1974). A comparison of a discriminant versus a clustering analysis of patient classification for chronic disease care. *Medical Care, 12*, 944–957.

Plummer, J. (1976). Patient classification proves staffing needs. *Dimensions in Health Services, 53*(5), 36–38.

Roehrl, P. K. (1979). Patient classification: a pilot test. *Supervisor Nurse, 10*(2), 21–27.

Rowland, H. S., & Rowland, B. L. (1980). *Nursing administration handbook.* Germantown, MD: Aspen Systems.

Simmons, D. A. (1980). *A classification scheme for client problems in community health nursing* (DHHS Publication No. HRA 8016). Washington DC: U.S. Government Printing Office.

Tilquin, C. (1976). Patient classification does work. *Dimensions in Health Services, 53*(1), 12–16.

Trivedi, V. M. (1979). Nursing judgment in selection of patient classification variables. *Research in Nursing and Health, 2*(3), 109–118.

Wolff, L., Weitzel, M. H., & Fuerst, E. (1979). *Fundamentals of nursing* (6th ed.). Philadelphia: Lippincott.

APPENDIX: EPISODE CODING FORM

	Begin
	Card 1
Agency_____	ID code __ __ 2 /01-03
Patient_____	_ID code___ ___ /04-05
	Episode number __ Card 1 /06-07
	(column 08 is left blank) /08

START OF EPISODE

	Response category					Don't know	Missing data	
Overall dependency	1	2	3	4		7	8	/09
Vision	1	2	3	4		7	8	/10
Hearing (w/aid if used)	1	2	3	4		7	8	/11
Expressive communication	1	2	3	4	5	7	8	/12
Receptive communication	1	2	3	4	5	7	8	/13
Bathing/showering	1	2	3			7	8	/14
Dressing	1	2	3			7	8	/15
Toileting	1	2	3			7	8	/16
Transferring (bed/chair)	1	2	3			7	8	/17
Continence	1	2	3	4		7	8	/18
Eating	1	2	3			7	8	/19
Walking	1	2	3			7	8	/20
Mobility	1	2	3	4		7	8	/21
Adaptive tasks	1	2	3			7	8	/22
Behavior problems	1	2	3			7	8	/23
Disorientation/memory impairment	1	2	3			7	8	/24
Mood disturbance	1	2				7	8	/25

	No	Yes	Missing data	
Income deficit	0	1	8	/26
Sanitation deficit	0	1	8	/27
Residence safety hazard	0	1	8	/28
Language barrier/dissatisfaction with services	0	1	8	/29
Social isolation	0	1	8	/30
Suspicious behavior pattern	0	1	8	/31
Compulsive behavior pattern	0	1	8	/32
Role change	0	1	8	/33
Interpersonal conflict	0	1	8	/34
Grief	0	1	8	/35
Confusion: attention span	0	1	8	/36

	No	Yes	MD	
Confusion: time, place, person	0	1	8	/37
Confusion: forgetfulness	0	1	8	/38
Feeling of hopelessness/worthlessness	0	1	8	/39
Excessive inward focus	0	1	8	/40
Expresses wish to die	0	1	8	/41
Fails to meet personal needs	0	1	8	/42
Feeling of appreciation	0	1	8	/43
Irritable	0	1	8	/44
Much purposeless activity	0	1	8	/45
Lacks caretaking skills	0	1	8	/46
Lacks consistent routine for caretaking	0	1	8	/47
Neglect	0	1	8	/48
Abuse	0	1	8	/49
Behavior inappropriate for age	0	1	8	/50
Hearing impairment	0	1	8	/51
Vision impairment	0	1	8	/52
Lacks ability to speak	0	1	8	/53
Inability to understand	0	1	8	/54
Relies on nonverbal communication	0	1	8	/55
Dentition impairment	0	1	8	/56
Abnormal breath patterns (SOB/dyspnea)	0	1	8	/57
Cough	0	1	8	/58
Cyanosis	0	1	8	/59
Noisy respiration	0	1	8	/60
Rhinorrhea	0	1	8	/61
Abnormal breath sounds	0	1	8	/62
Edema	0	1	8	/63
Cramping/pain in extremities	0	1	8	/64
Decreased pulses	0	1	8	/65
Discoloration of skin/cyanosis	0	1	8	/66
Temp. change affected area	0	1	8	/67
Varicosities	0	1	8	/68
Fainting/syncopal episodes	0	1	8	/69
Abnormal blood pressure	0	1	8	/70
Pulse deficit	0	1	8	/71
Irregular heart rate	0	1	8	/72
Excessive rapid/slow heart rate	0	1	8	/73
Reports anginal pain	0	1	8	/74
Abnormal heart sounds	0	1	8	/75
Limited ROM/contractures	0	1	8	/76
Poor coordination	0	1	8	/77
Gait/ambulation disturbance	0	1	8	/78

(Column 79 is left blank) /79

Episode data code E /80

Agency ID __ __ 2   **Patient ID __ __**   **Episode __ __ 2**

Begin Card 2 /01-07

(column 08 is left blank)   /08

	No	Yes	MD	
				/09
Decreased muscle strength/muscle tightness	0	1	8	/10
Inability to manage ADL	0	1	8	/11
Tremors	0	1	8	/12
Nausea/vomiting	0	1	8	/13
Difficulty chewing/swallowing	0	1	8	/14
Indigestion/heartburn	0	1	8	/15
Anorexia	0	1	8	/16
Anemia	0	1	8	/17
Abnormal weight loss	0	1	8	/18
Inability to cope with body changes	0	1	8	/19
Lifestyle incongruent with physiological changes	0	1	8	/20
Diarrhea	0	1	8	/21
Constipation	0	1	8	/22
Pain with defecation	0	1	8	/23
Minimal bowel sounds	0	1	8	/24
Blood in stool	0	1	8	/25
Abnormal colon	0	1	8	
Cramping/abdominal discomfort	0	1	8	/26
Increased frequency of stools	0	1	8	/27
Incontinent of stools	0	1	8	/28
Incontinent of urine	0	1	8	/29
Urgency/frequency of stools	0	1	8	/30
Burning/painful urination	0	1	8	/31
Inability to empty bladder	0	1	8	/32
Nocturia	0	1	8	/33
Polyuria	0	1	8	/34
Oliguria	0	1	8	/35
Hematuria	0	1	8	/36
Lesion (wound/burn/incision)	0	1	8	/37
Rash	0	1	8	/38
Inflammation	0	1	8	/39
Drainage	0	1	8	/40
Pain: client statement	0	1	8	/41
Pain: elevated pulse, respiration, BP	0	1	8	/42
Pain: compensatory movement	0	1	8	/43
Pain: pallor, sweating	0	1	8	/44
Lacks response to normal stimuli	0	1	8	/45
Abnormal intake of essential food/fluids	0	1	8	/46
Emaciated/obese	0	1	8	/47

	No	Yes		MD	
Awakens frequently	0	1		8	/48
Insufficient rest/sleep	0	1		8	/49
Sedentary lifestyle	0	1		8	/50
Inappropriate exercise	0	1		8	/51
Personal hygiene deficit	0	1		8	/52
Substance misuse	0	1		8	/53
Noncompliance with medical visits	0	1		8	/54
Noncompliance with Rx	0	1		8	/55
Fails to obtain necessary equipment	0	1	8	/56	
Deviates from prescribed dosage	0	1		8	/57
Lacks system for taking medications	0	1		8	/58
Medications improperly stored	0	1		8	/59
Does not obtain med refill	0	1		8	/60
Unable to integrate diet into balanced nutrition	0	1		8	/61
Does not adhere to diet Rx	0	1		8	/62
Unable to demonstrate/relate procedure accurately	0	1		8	/63
Requires nursing skill					
Unable to perform procedure without assistance	0	1		8	/64
Unable to operate special equipment correctly	0	1		8	/66

(columns 67–79 are left blank) /67-79

Episode data code **E**   /80

**Begin
Card 3**

Agency ID __ __ 2   **Patient ID**__ __   **Episode** __ __ 3 /01-07

(column 08 is left blank)   /08

END OF EPISODE

	Response category					DK	MD	
Overall dependency	1	2	3	4		7	8	/09

Length of episode (days) __ __ __ /10-12

Reason for discharge	recovered 1	/13
	stable condition 2	
	financial problems 3	
	acutely ill 4	
	deceased 5	
	moved out of area 6	
	other 7	
	missing data 8	

Disposition at D/C own care .... 1 /14

family care 2

residential care 3

nursing home 4

hospital 5

moved out of area 6

other services 7

missing data 8

Primary diagnosis __ __ __ /15-17

Second diagnosis __ __ __ Third diagnosis __ __ __ /18-23

(columns 24-25 are left blank) /24-25

	No	Yes	MD	
Income deficit	0	1	8	/26
Sanitation deficit	0	1	8	/27
Residence safety hazard	0	1	8	/28
Language barrier/dissatisfied with services	0	1	8	/29
Social isolation	0	1	8	/30
Suspicious behavior pattern	0	1	8	/31
Compulsive behavior pattern	0	1	8	/32
Role change	0	1	8	/33
Interpersonal conflict	0	1	8	/34
Grief	0	1	8	/35
Confusion/attention span	0	1	8	/36
Confusion/time, place, person	0	1	8	/37
Confusion/forgetfulness	0	1	8	/38
Feeling of hopelessness/worthlessness	0	1	8	/39
Excessive inward focus	0	1	8	/40
Expresses wish to die	0	1	8	/41
Fails to meet personal needs	0	1	8	/42
Feeling of apprehension	0	1	8	/43
Irritable	0	1	8	/44
Much purposeless activity	0	1	8	/45
Lacks caretaking skills	0	1	8	/46
Lacks consistent routine for caretaking	0	1	8	/47
Neglect	0	1	8	/48
Abuse	0	1	8	/49
Behavior inappropriate for age	0	1	8	/50
Hearing impairment	0	1	8	/51
Vision impairment	0	1	8	/52
Lacks ability to speak	0	1	8	/53
Inability to understand	0	1	8	/54
Relies on nonverbal communication	0	1	8	/55
Dentition impairment	0	1	8	/56
Abnormal breath patterns (SOB/dyspnea)	0	1	8	/57

	No	Yes	MD	
Cough	0	1	8	/58
Cyanosis	0	1	8	/59
Noisy respiration	0	1	8	/60
Rhinorrhea	0	1	8	/61
Abnormal breath sounds	0	1	8	/62
Edema	0	1	8	/63
Cramping/pain in extremities	0	1	8	/64
Decreased pulses	0	1	8	/65
Discoloration of skin/cyanosis	0	1	8	/66
Temp. change affected area	0	1	8	/67
Varicosities	0	1	8	/68
Fainting/syncopal episodes	0	1	8	/69
Abnormal blood pressure	0	1	8	/70
Pulse deficit	0	1	8	/71
Irregular heart rate	0	1	8	/72
Excessive rapid/slow heart rate	0	1	8	/73
Reports anginal pain	0	1	8	/74
Abnormal heart sounds	0	1	8	/75
Limited ROM/contractures	0	1	8	/76
Poor coordination	0	1	8	/77
Gait/ambulation disturbance	0	1	8	/78

(column 79 is left blank)   /79
Episode data code E   /80

Begin Card 4

Agency ID __ __ 2   **Patient ID__ __**   **Episode __ __ 4** /01-07
(column 08 is left blank)   /08
(column 08 is left blank)   /08

	No	Yes	MD	
Decreased muscle strength/ muscle tightness	0	1	8	/09
Inability to manage ADL	0	1	8	/10
Tremors	0	1	8	/11
Nausea/vomiting	0	1	8	/12
Difficulty chewing/swallowing	0	1	8	/13
Indigestion/heartburn	0	1	8	/14
Anorexia	0	1	8	/15
Anemia	0	1	8	/16
Abnormal weight loss	0	1	8	/17
Inability to cope with body changes	0	1	8	/18
Lifestyle incongruent with physiological changes	0	1	8	/19

	No	Yes	MD	
Diarrhea	0	1	8	/20
Constipation	0	1	8	/21
Pain with defecation	0	1	8	/22
Minimal bowel sounds	0	1	8	/23
Blood in stool	0	1	8	/24
Abnormal colon	0	1	8	/25
Cramping/abdominal discomfort	0	1	8	/26
Increased frequency of stools	0	1	8	/27
Incontinent of stools	0	1	8	/28
Incontinent of urine	0	1	8	/29
Urgency/frequency	0	1	8	/30
Burning/painful urination	0	1	8	/31
Inability to empty bladder	0	1	8	/32
Nocturia	0	1	8	/33
Polyuria	0	1	8	/34
Oliguria	0	1	8	/35
Hematuria	0	1	8	/36
Lesion (wound/burn/incision)	0	1	8	/37
Rash	0	1	8	/38
Inflammation	0	1	8	/39
Drainage	0	1	8	/40
Pain: client statement	0	1	8	/41
Pain: elevated pulse, respiration, BP	0	1	8	/42
Pain: compensatory movement	0	1	8	/43
Pain: pallor, sweating	0	1	8	/44
Lacks response to normal stimuli	0	1	8	/45
Abnormal intake of essential food/fluids	0	1	8	/46
Emaciated/obese	0	1	8	/47
Awakens frequently	0	1	8	/48
Insufficient rest/sleep	0	1	8	/49
Sedentary lifestyle	0	1	8	/50
Inappropriate exercise	0	1	8	/51
Personal hygiene deficit	0	1	8	/52
Substance misuse	0	1	8	/53
Noncompliance with medical visits	0	1	8	/54
Noncompliance with Rx	0	1	8	/55
Fails to obtain necessary equipment	0	1	8	/56
Deviates from prescribed dosage	0	1	8	/57
Lacks system for taking medications	0	1	8	/58
Medications improperly stored	0	1	8	/59
Does not obtain med refills	0	1	8	/60
Unable to integrate diet into balanced nutrition	0	1	8	/61
Does not adhere to diet Rx	0	1	8	/62

	No	Yes	MD	
Unable to demonstrate/relate procedure accurately	0	1	8	/63
Requires nursing skill	0	1	8	/64
Unable to perform procedure without assistance	0	1	8	/65
Unable to operate special equipment correctly	0	1	8	/66

(columns 67–79 is left blank) /67–79

Episode data code E /80

20

The Individualized Care Index

Gwen van Servellen

This chapter discusses the Individualized Care Index, a measure of the extent to which nurses individualize their care of patients.

PURPOSE

The concept of individualized care is frequently alluded to in professional nursing literature in descriptions of quality patient care. It is addressed both as the process by which high levels of quality care and patient satisfaction are achieved and as the outcome of selected nursing care modalities such as primary nursing in a hospital setting. Initial studies were undertaken to establish the discriminate validity of the Individualized Care Index (ICI)-Survey Format and are reported here. Background on the reliability and validity assessments of the Individualized Care Index will be discussed. The survey to measure nurses' performance of individualized care practices in an inpatient setting is included. This survey was used in a comparative study of registered nurse responses to the frequency with which they perform individualized care when their inpatient hospital units are organized around team, total patient care, or primary nursing modalities. The results of this study are discussed. Finally, additional versions of the original survey are available to assess specific nurse–patient interactions and are designed as both patient and nurse surveys. Implications of the use of the ICI in its present form is discussed along with indications for future tests of validity and reliability.

CONCEPTUAL BASIS

Individualized nursing care translates all standardized nursing procedures and activities in terms of the uniqueness of each patient situation (Marram, Barrett, & Bevis, 1974, 1979). Individualized care can also be said to include patient-centered communicative responses where concern for patients' thoughts or problems is expressed and a willingness to listen and to stimulate patients' self-care potential is provided (Chapman, 1977). High levels of individualized nursing care are reported to be both an outcome of a nursing care modality (primary nursing) and the process by which high levels of patient satisfaction and quality care are achieved.

As early as 1961, individualized approaches to nursing care were advocated (Abdellah, 1961). The essential element of patient-centered nursing care is seen as the individualization of the nursing approach to the patient's needs. The concept of individualized care also emerged in descriptions of the nursing process and quality patient care. An essential of nursing education is to motivate nurses to think in terms of each individual patient (Yura & Walsh, 1973). Subsequent to these endorsements, it was used in descriptions of patients' bills of rights and was associated with the achievement of quality patient care (Haussman, Hegyvary, & Newman, 1976; Johnson & Tingey, 1976) and patient satisfaction (Hinshaw, Gerber, Atwood, & Allen, 1983). In addition, the concept is intimately linked with primary nursing, a nursing care modality that has been considered and implemented by large numbers of hospitals both in the United States (van Servellen, 1980) and overseas (Hegyvary, 1982). In various pilot studies conducted by Marram, Flynn, Abaravich, and Carey (1976) and van Servellen (1980) it was found that greater numbers of individualized care behaviors on the part of the nurse were perceived by patients on primary nursing units compared to patients on those units practicing team and functional nursing. Furthermore, it was suggested that greater levels of individualized care may be a distinguishing facet of this mode of organizing care in a hospital setting.

The following is an outline of the steps taken over a 2–year period to refine and test the Individualized Care Index (ICI). Included is a review of the steps that have occurred to date and a detailed discussion of a test of discriminate validity. The issues of validity as well as reliability (measure of internal consistency) are discussed.

PROCEDURES FOR ICI

The first step in designing the measure was to establish a valid definition of the concept. The initial content validity of the ICI was assured by establishing a list of individualized care behaviors by three means: a review of the literature, the input of a panel of judges, and an initial pretest.

An extensive review of the literature dating back to 1960 was conducted. The concept of individualized care, as well as various related phenomena, was explored: patient-centered care, comprehensive care, and coordinated-continuous patient care delivery. It was believed that these concepts may not be independent of one another and may form a cluster of related phenomena.

A panel of judges, which consisted of three graduate faculty and two graduate students, was asked to review a list of nursing care behaviors generated from the literature by the researcher and research assistants. They were asked to complete two tasks: (1) to differentiate those behaviors judged to be individualized care behaviors from irrelevant and bureaucratic care behaviors, and (2) to classify the individualized care items, if they could, according to the following categories: patient-centered care, comprehensive care, coordinated care, and continuity of care. In addition, each member was asked to alter the items to make them clearer and more precise. An analysis of the nursing care behaviors revealed that 64 of 80 individualized care items were judged to be individualized care actions.

This complete list of behaviors was subjected to another validity test, in which a larger group of nurses was asked to judge the items for their representativeness. A sample of 41 graduate students who were practicing as part-time staff nurses was asked to rate each item on a 5–point Likert-type scale. They were asked to judge how well each behavior fit their concept of individualized care, with 5 = *Strongly agree* and 1 = *Strongly disagree.* Of the initial full 80 nursing care items, 55 were perceived to be individualized care actions with mean scores of 4.0 and above. Initial items were reviewed for redundancy and overlap. The final selected items were subjected to further analysis and resulted in the design of the ICI—Survey of Nurse Performance of Individualized Care (see Appendix: Performance of Nursing Actions survey) which consists of 45 items and includes three individualized care factors: patient-centered comprehensive care, patient-centered coordinated care, and patient-centered inquiry/assessment.

DESCRIPTION

The purpose of the ICI-Survey of Nurse Performance of Individualized Care is to measure the extent to which nurses individualize their care to their patients. Its subscales allow the researcher to differentiate among categories of individualized care to learn which are practiced at greater or lesser frequency.

The ICI-Survey of Nurse Performance of Individualized Care consists of two sections; the first section is a set of 11 questions derived from the American Nurses' Association (1981) *Inventory of Registered Nurses,* aimed at obtaining key demographic information about the respondents. The second section, consisting of 45 questions, elicits responses about the frequency with which nurses perceive themselves as fulfilling each of 29 discrete individualized care nursing actions for their patients as well other nursing behaviors. For example, how frequently do you ask patients what they would like to know about their illness and discuss with patients the care that is planned for them while they are in the hospital? Nurses are asked to respond to a five–point rating scale, as follows: <u>with *none* of my patients</u> = 1 and <u>with *all* of my patients</u> = 5. An additional 13 items from the Qualpacs instrument (Wandelt & Ager, 1974) and three items addressing indirect aspects of care were included to mask the intent of the questionnaire, which focused heavily on patient-centered interactions of the nurse–patient dyad. These additional items included such behaviors as "Make decisions that reflect knowledge of facts and good judgment" and "Communicate clearly ideas, facts, and concepts about the patient in charting." A social desirability response pattern was expected to influence the respondent's answers. Hinshaw (personal communication, June, 1984) suggests that in relationship to the Measurements of Clinical and Educational Nursing Outcomes Projects, such a subset of quality nursing care items, if included, could mask the intent or essence of the study.

The ICI is a survey addressed specifically to registered nurses who deliver direct patient care in an inpatient hospital setting. Procedures for administering the survey include the following steps. The sample of RNs should be identified. The researcher may either survey the behaviors of all RNs on particular nursing units or sample randomly from these units or the hospital as a whole. The ICI can yield an overall estimate of individualized care practices at the unit level or be used to identify weaknesses in the practice of individual nurses. Because it is a self-report measure and may not accurately reflect nursing practices, it is advised that additional data, for example, from patient reports of nurses' actions, be incorporated in an analysis of nurses' performances of individualized care. A patient report version of the instrument is available from the author. Additionally, an alternative form of the ICI Performance of Nursing Actions, evaluating individualized care behaviors, has been developed that asks the nurse to identify those behaviors performed for a specific patient.

Scoring of the ICI requires the researcher to calculate the mean score and standard deviation for each respondent on each subscale of the ICI as well as on the ICI as a whole. All items are assigned an equal weight. Interpretation of the scores is based on judging scores as "high" or "low" given the average score of the nurse population under study.

RELIABILITY AND VALIDITY

Reliability of the ICI was determined by two means: a test–retest measure and a measure of internal consistency.

A test–retest procedure was used with a preliminary pilot test of the instrument. The ICI was administered to 10 students. Its reliability was estimated by a test–retest trial in which a correlation coefficient of .86 was found when these students were tested 1 week later.

A measure of internal consistency of items using Cronbach's alpha was undertaken with a sample of 838 practicing RNs in 18 hospitals. Cronbach's alpha was calculated for each factor in the ICI: patient-centered comprehensive care, patient-centered coordinated care, and patient-centered inquiry/assessment. Cronbach's alpha, calculated from the average interitem correlation, is interpreted as a measure of the reliability of each factor (Carmines & Zeller, 1969). The interitem correlations were only moderate: Factor I, .56; Factor II, .35; and Factor III, .49. Each subscale, however, had an acceptable alpha coefficient: Factor I, .91; Factor II, .85; and Factor III, .91. These alpha values indicate good reliability for each factor considered as a sum of ratings for its items.

Tests of the validity of the ICI were undertaken with two separate studies: one measuring the construct validity of the ICI, and another, its discriminate validity. Particular detailed attention will be given to the test of discriminate validity, as it represents the latest study utilizing the ICI.

The construct validity of the ICI items was the focus of a study of a large sample of RNs practicing nursing in a hospital setting. The purpose of this study was to employ a factor analytic procedure to identify the specific subdimensions of the ICI. A ratio of 10 respondents for each item set the outer limits for sampling RNs for this phase of the research. The factor analytic procedure was employed to accomplish two things: (1) to reveal the underlying dimensionality of the concept and (2) to provide a valid means of reducing a large set of items to a smaller representative set of indices. The ICI was administered to 838 practicing RNs in 19 randomly selected hospitals.

Because of skew of the distributions of the nursing behavior item ratings, the conventional factor analysis assuming normal distributions is not applicable. Therefore, it was decided to dichotomize the distributions at a value of 4 (> 4 vs. < 4) and to employ Muthen's (1981) two-procedure factor analysis for dichotomous variables. The first procedure is an exploratory factor analysis that enables one to determine the number of factors present and to form hypotheses regarding factor structure. The second procedure is a confirmatory analysis that tests the goodness of fit of a model for which one specifies both the number of factors and the items (nursing behaviors) that have loadings on each of the factors.

Results of the exploratory factor analysis were the following. Of the 80 items (excluding five nonsense items) 44 items were selected as most useful to determine subfactors of individualized care. The criterion for selecting these items was that they showed sufficient variability in ratings to provide useful information on subjects' differing perceptions of nursing behavior. Results of the exploratory factor analysis indicated that four factors could be differentiated: a bureaucratic factor and a three-factor individualized care model. The individualized care factors were composed of 29 discrete items, two of which loaded >.40 on two factors. These factors were interpreted and categorized as follows: Factor I: Patient-centered coordinated care (11 items); Factor II: Patient-centered comprehensive care (10 items); and Factor III: Patient-centered inquiry/assessment (10 items).

Finally, a test of discriminate validity was conducted to examine the ability of the ICI to distinguish between different modalities of nursing care that were purported to yield lower or higher levels of individualized care. Greater numbers of certain patient-centered expressive care behaviors were found in a study of a primary nursing setting compared to a total patient care setting. It was hypothesized that nurses' performance of individualized care behavior (as measured by the ICI) will vary, depending on the modality practiced.

The hypotheses of the study were:

> Nurses' performance of individualized care behaviors (as measured by the ICI Survey Format) will be significantly higher for primary nursing staff than for total patient care and team nursing staff.
> Nurses' performance of individualized care behaviors (as measured by the ICI Survey Format) will be significantly higher for total patient care than for team nursing staff.

Performance of individualized care was defined as nurses' self-reported frequency with which they performed nursing actions specified in the ICI.

Three nursing care modalities were compared. These were team nursing, total patient care, and primary nursing. Each modality was seen to have a distinct method of nurse–patient assignment. For the purpose of this study these modalities were defined in the following manner.

Team nursing—An RN and aide and/or LVN are assigned to a group of patients, usually 12 to 15. The RN team leader administers medications and treatments; the LVN and/or aide completes other aspects of care for these 12 to 15 patients.

Total patient care—Nurses are assigned to 4 to 7 patients for whom they deliver total patient care. These nurses may be RNs or LVNs; however, their care (on a single shift) is not supplemented by another nurse or aide. There is no expectation that the same nurse(s) when on duty will be reassigned the same patients.

Primary nursing—Nurses are assigned to 4 to 7 patients for whom they deliver total patient care. Nurses are designated as primary nurses or associate nurses. However, only RNs can be primary nurses; associate nurses can be either RNs or LVNs and can care for the patient when the primary nurse is not on duty. There is an expectation that primary nurses will be reassigned to the same patients throughout these patients' hospitalization.

Continuity is a measure that can be assigned to a unit as a whole and represents the average rate that nurses are assigned to care for the same patient. By definition these modalities differ in the extent that continuity of the nurse–patient relationship is upheld. A secondary hypothesis was that different levels of continuity will be observed across modalities. For the purpose of this study, average continuity rate represented the proportion of time the nurse on duty has been assigned to the same patient from the day of admission.

SAMPLE AND SETTING

A systematic sampling of nursing units in randomly selected hospitals was used for this study. Using the criteria of 200 beds and Joint Commission for the Accreditation of Hospitals accreditation, a sample of eight hospitals was randomly drawn from the American Hospital Association (1983) hospital listings, using a table of random numbers. The sampling criteria for choosing units from participating hospitals were as follows: (1) the unit should service largely general medical-surgical patients and (2) the unit had to practice one of the following three modalities: team nursing, total patient care, or primary nursing, as previously defined. A double-level screening process was conducted to choose appropriate units. Directors of nursing in these hospitals were asked to select units that met these criteria; then head nurses on these units were asked to verify these judgments by completing a head nurse survey. The survey asked for clarification about staffing patterns, assignments of staff to patients, and the role of the staff RN in caring for patients.

A total of 11 hospital units were chosen to participate. Of these units three were primary nursing units; four, team nursing; and four, total patient care units. The objective of sampling RNs from these units was to enlist all consenting RNs to complete the survey. A minimum of 80% of the total RN staff on each unit was required if the unit was to remain in the study.

A survey was delivered to each RN by the head nurse on the unit. The surveys, enclosed in sealed envelopes, were returned to a large manila envelope on the unit, addressed to the researcher, and subsequently picked up by the researcher two weeks from the day of distribution.

Customary procedures to protect the rights of human subjects were utilized. Nurses were informed of their rights and signed a consent form to participate in the study.

A total of 164 nurses were surveyed in 11 hospital units of eight hospitals. The sample breakdown was the following: Team nursing, 55; total patient care, 53; and primary nursing, 56.

The majority of the nurses surveyed (95.1%) were female; the median age range was 35 to 39 years. Nearly two thirds (105, or 64%) of the sample were Caucasian; the next most common ethnicity and the only other group represented in significant numbers was Asian (43, or 26.2%). The basic RN preparation included 44.5% from AA programs, 27.4% from diploma programs, and 27.4% from BSN programs. When highest level of nursing education was considered, nurses graduating from AA programs were still greatest in number: 40.9% had attained an AA degree; 25.6%, a diploma; and 31.1%, a BSN/BS degree. Only two nurses held MN or MSN degrees. The majority worked full-time (79.3%), were career appointments (76.2%), and were considered permanent staff (83.5%). The majority also worked 8–hour shifts, either days (37.8%) or evenings (34.1%). As for their area of specialization, all nurses worked in medical-surgical nursing; 29.3% worked in a combination of medical-surgical services (e.g., medical and oncology or medical-general/surgery). Sixty-four percent of the sample had less than 10 years of nursing experience; the median range was 5 to 10 years. In comparison, 14.4% of the sample had less than 10 years hospital nursing experience, and the median range was 3 to 5 years.

INDIVIDUALIZED CARE AS A FUNCTION OF NURSING CARE MODALITY

The primary hypothesis of interest is this study was that nurses' performance of individualized care behaviors (as measured by the ICI) would vary across nursing care modalities. Results should indicate a low level for staff practicing team nursing to a high level for staff practicing primary nursing, with staff practicing total patient care (TPC) somewhere in between. Although the data indicated a trend in the expected direction for the average total ICI scores, this result was not statistically significant. This lack of a significant difference in the total ICI scores among the three nursing modalities held for each of the three ICI subdimensions.

It was also of interest to determine if differences in the demographic makeup of the staff had any effect on the relationship between modality and the performance of individualized care. The data failed to indicate any significant differences in the average total ICI scores between modalities when controlling for education (basic as well as higher), area of nursing (e.g., surgical), and number of years practiced (in general as well as exclusively as an RN in a hospital setting). There was also no evidence that education, area of nursing, or length of experience in themselves had a significant effect on the reported level of individualized care practiced.

As would be expected, night nurses practiced individualized care differently from either day or evening nurses. There was a statistically significant difference in the average total overall ICI scores between nurses on days and evenings (X = 112 + 13 and 112 + 14, respectively) and nurses on nights (X = 100 + 17). Results of a one-way analysis of variance (ANOVA) indicated an F-ratio of 9.96 (df = 2,159, p = .0001).

Due to sample size constraints, only Caucasians and Asians were used in analyzing the effect of ethnicity on reported practice of individualized care behaviors. There was a statistically significant difference in the average total overall ICI score among the three nursing modalities when taking into account differences in ethnicity results of a two-way ANOVA F-ratio of 3–3 (df = 2,140, p = .04). The trend in individualized care behaviors expected (see statement of primary hypotheses) is most evident in Asian nurses. Specifically, Asian nurses practicing team nursing have a significantly lower average total overall ICI score than Asian nurses practicing total patient care (TPC) (p = .03) and primary nursing (p = .02). Caucasian nurses practicing primary nursing appear to perform more individualized care behaviors than Caucasian nurses practicing TPC (p = .04). Asian nurses had a lower average ICI score than Caucasian nurses when practicing team nursing but this relationship was reversed for Asian nurses practicing TPC and primary nursing. Thus, it appears that ethnicity of the nurse is not only an important factor to take into account when assessing individualized care within a given nursing modality but that the pattern of individualized care behavior across nursing modalities varies depending on the ethnic background of the nurse.

As indicated previously, a secondary purpose of the study was to examine the continuity of care on each unit to determine how well these units practiced a single modality. Continuity of care was measured in two ways: average and corrected continuity. Although the expected relationship between average continuity and modality was evident (i.e., lower continuity for team nursing to higher continuity for primary nursing), it is of interest to note that this trend was not apparent when continuity was measured by corrected continuity, which was thought to be a better measure than average continuity.

CONCLUSIONS AND RECOMMENDATIONS

The overall aim of this program of research was to establish the validity and reliability of the ICI-Survey Format. The specific purpose of the most recent study was to test the discriminant validity of the ICI with nurses practicing in different nursing care modalities.

The general implications of the reliability and validity assessments indicate that the ICI should undergo further tests of validity and reliability. As was noted, the ICI could not discriminate among nursing care modalities. This fact could be related to more than one phenomenon. First, the nursing care modalities may not have been sufficiently different to reveal differences in performance. One should also consider that the results may be due to the self-report nature of the tool. Observations of nursing behaviors may be the best approach to measuring this variable. Of significance here was that the researcher's communications with head nurses suggested that no modality was practiced in its pure form. Primary nursing units had difficulty preserving the continuity of nurse–patient relationship, and team nursing units sometimes did TPC with selected patients, for example, medical-oncology patients. Also, TPC units were sometimes low on RN staff and employed a mini-team arrangement and in still other instances used a primary nursing mode, when staffing permitted, with selected patients. The fact that these modalities were probably not discretely different was also evident in the analysis of continuity of assignment and nursing care modality. Continuity of care should be strongly related to modality, and the lack of a strong relationship could explain, in part, why the relationship between modality and individualized care was not strongly evident. That is, it is further evidence that the modalities were not practiced in a pure enough form. This, obviously, would make it difficult for the ICI to discriminate among the modalities.

ACKNOWLEDGMENTS

This study was funded in part by an Academic Senate Grant from the University of California, Los Angeles. Recognition is given to Dr. Noel Wheeler, PhD, Director of Statistics/Biomathematic Consulting Clinic, and Ms. Sarah Forsythe, MS, statistician, UCLA, for their assistance in the data analysis.

REFERENCES

Abdellah, F. (1961). *Patient-centered approaches to nursing.* New York: Macmillan.

American Hospital Association (1983). *American Hospital Association guide to the health care field.* Chicago: Author.

American Nurses' Association (1981). *Inventory of registered nurses.* Kansas City MO: Author.

Carmines, E., & Zeller, R. (1979). *Reliability and validity assessment.* Beverly Hills, CA: Sage.

Chapman, J. (1977). Effects of different nursing approaches upon selected postoperative responses of male herniorrhaphy patients. In F. Downs & M. Newman (Eds.), *A source book of nursing research* (2nd ed.), (pp. 15–23). Philadelphia: F. A. Davis.

Haussmann, R. K. D., Hegyvary, S. T., & Newman, J. F. (1976). *Monitoring quality of nursing care: II. Assessment and study of correlates* (DHEW Publication No. (HRA) 76–7). Bethesda, MD: Department of Health, Education and Welfare.

Hegyvary, S. (1982). *The change to primary nursing—a cross cultural view of professional nursing practice.* St. Louis: Mosby.

Hinshaw, A. S., Gerber, R. M., Atwood, J. R., & Allen, J. R. (1983). The use of predictive modeling to test nursing practice outcomes. *Nursing Research, 33*(1), 35–42.

Johnson, G. V., & Tingey, S. (1976). Matrix organization: Blueprint of nursing care organization for the 80s. *Hospital and Health Services Administration, 21,* 27–39.

Marram, G., Barrett, M., & Bevis, E. (1974). *Primary nursing—A model for individualized care.* St. Louis: Mosby.

Marram, G., Barrett, M., & Bevis, E. (1979). *Primary nursing—A model for individualized care* (2nd ed.). St. Louis: Mosby.

Marram G., Flynn, K., Abaravich, W., & Carey, C. (1976). *Cost-effectiveness of primary and team nursing.* Wakefield, MA: Contemporary Publishing.

Muthen, B. (1981). Factor analysis of dichotomous variables. In E. Borgatta & D.J. Jackson (Eds.), *Factor analysis and measurement in sociological research: a multidimensional perspective* (p. 85). San Francisco: Sage.

van Servellen, G. (1980). Primary nursing—The adoption of a nursing care modality. *Nursing and Health Care, 1*(3), 144–150.

van Servellen, G. (1988). The Individualized Care Index . In C. F. Waltz & O. L. Strickland (Eds.), *Measurement of nursing outcomes: Vol. 1: Measuring client outcomes* (pp. 499–522). New York: Springer Publishing Co.

Wandelt, M., & Ager, J. (1974). *Quality Patient Care Scale.* New York: Appleton, Century & Crofts.

Yura, H., & Walsh, M. (1973). *The nursing process—Assessing, planning, implementing, evaluating* (2nd ed.). New York: Appleton-Century-Crofts.

APPENDIX: PERFORMANCE OF NURSING ACTIONS

Nurses complete many tasks in caring for patients. Some of these tasks may be performed more frequently than others. You are asked to judge how frequently you do these things by indicating the proportion of patients for whom you complete these activities. That is, how frequently do you perform these behaviors in the administration of nursing care to the patients to whom you are assigned?

Choice 1: With none of my patients
Choice 2: With a few of my patients
Choice 3: With some of my patients
Choice 4: With most of my patients
Choice 5: With all of my patients

Circle the answer that best reflects your judgment.

	With none of my patients	With a few of my patients	With some of my patients	With most of my patients	With all of my patients
1. Discuss with the family what role they would like to assume in providing care for patient while he/she is in the hospital.	1	2	3	4	5
2. Give patients an opportunity to explain their feelings.	1	2	3	4	5
3. Meet with the oncoming shift to discuss the patient's problems.	1	2	3	4	5
4. Sit down with patients to discuss their care.	1	2	3	4	5
5. Make sure patients know what roles physicians will play in their care.	1	2	3	4	5
6. Allow the patients time to talk about their fears or concerns.	1	2	3	4	5
7. Meet patient's daily hygiene needs for cleanliness.	1	2	3	4	5
8. Discuss with patients the care that is planned for them while they are in the hospital.	1	2	3	4	5
9. After completing the nursing assessment, validate with the patient what you have identified as his/her problems.	1	2	3	4	5
10. Discuss with the dietitian theh diet plan for the patient.	1	2	3	4	5

	With none of my patients	With a few of my patients	With some of my patients	With most of my patients	With all of my patients
11. Allow patients to assume as much responsibility for their own care as they can.	1	2	3	4	5
12. Make sure patients understand who will be taking care of them.	1	2	3	4	5
13. Ask patients what they would like to know about their illness.	1	2	3	4	5
14. Ask patients if they have any preferences about any aspect of their care.	1	2	3	4	5
15. Allow patients to set the times for their activities and treatments as much as possible, e.g., baths, medications, bedtime.	1	2	3	4	5
16. Help patients accept dependence/ independence (as appropriate to their condition).	1	2	3	4	5
17. Find out if the patient has ever talked with anyone who has the same illness.	1	2	3	4	5
18. Participate in conference concerning your patients' care.	1	2	3	4	5
19. Take action to meet the patient's need for adequate hydration and elimination.	1	2	3	4	5
20. Adapt expected patient activities to the physical and mental capabilities of the patient.	1	2	3	4	5
21. Make sure patients know the names of the persons responsible for specific procedures and/or treatments.	1	2	3	4	5
22. Include the patient's family in planning the patient's care upon discharge.	1	2	3	4	5
23. Make sure patients understand about their medications, such as reason why and side effects.	1	2	3	4	5
24. Write 24-hr nursing orders for the patient on the care plan.	1	2	3	4	5
25. Support patients in learning about their care.	1	2	3	4	5
26. Talk with patients about what they know about their illness.	1	2	3	4	5

	With none of my patients	With a few of my patients	With some of my patients	With most of my patients	With all of my patients
27. Review the information that you gave the patient to be sure that he/she understood.	1	2	3	4	5
28. Carry out medical and surgical asepsis during treatments and special procedures.	1	2	3	4	5
29. Approach patients in a kind, gentle, and friendly manner.	1	2	3	4	5
30. Discuss with patients the impact their hospitalization will have on their lives and families.	1	2	3	4	5
31. Complete all "hands on" nursing procedures for the patient with skill and sensitivity to patient needs.	1	2	3	4	5
32. Keep informed of your patients' condition and whereabouts during your assigned shifts.	1	2	3	4	5
33. Ask patients what their usual daily activities are, such as work, hobbies and recreation.	1	2	3	4	5
34. Report the pertinent incidents of the patient's behavior during interaction with other staff.	1	2	3	4	5
35. Protect patient's sensitivities and rights to privacy.	1	2	3	4	5
36. Through talking with patients and/or their families, determine what nursing care needs patients have that are different from the expected or anticipated needs.	1	2	3	4	5
37. Inform the doctor that you are the patient's nurse.	1	2	3	4	5
38. Ask patients if they have any questions about their care.	1	2	3	4	5
39. Give patients explanations and verbal reassurances when needed.	1	2	3	4	5
40. Ask patients if they understood all the things that their physician has told them.	1	2	3	4	5
41. Communicate clearly ideas, facts, and concepts about the patient in charting.	1	2	3	4	5

	With none of my patients	With a few of my patients	With some of my patients	With most of my patients	With all of my patients
42. Make sure that changes in care and the care plans for your patients reflect the continuous evaluation of nursing care given.	1	2	3	4	5
43. Make decisions that reflect knowledge of facts and good judgment.	1	2	3	4	5
44. Assess the patient's emotional state frequently.	1	2	3	4	5
45. Discuss with patients how their illness will affect them and their family.	1	2	3	4	5

21

Manifestations of Early Recognition: A Measure of Nursing Expertise

Ptlene Minick

This chapter discusses the Manifestations of Early Recognition Scale, a measure of attributes associated with the skill of the early recognition of patient problems.

PURPOSE

The early recognition of patient problems is a particularly important skill of acute care nurses because with interventions, early problems are less likely to progress to major complications. Many investigators have found expertise and keen assessment skills associated with personal attributes of nurses (Benner, Hooper-Kyriakidis, & Stannard, 1999; Benner & Wrubel, 1989; Hamers, Huijer Abu Saad, & Halfens, 1994; Jenny & Logan, 1992; Minick, 1995; Minick & Harvey, in press). Attributes associated specifically with the skills of early recognition include knowing and caring, along with a willingness to take risks for the patient/family and an ethical commitment to be the "good nurse" (Minick, 1995; Minick & Harvey, in press).

CONCEPTUAL FRAMEWORK

Findings from three phenomenological studies provided the conceptual basis for instrument development. A total of 50 critical care and medical-surgical nurses participated in either group or individual interviews. Nursing experience of the participants ranged from six months to 32 years with a mean of 15.2 years. Interviews lasted from 20 to 90 minutes. The question used to guide the interviews was, "Tell me about a time when you felt you made a difference with a patient. It could be something simple that you might do every day with many patients . . . . or it may focus more toward the family than the patient." Verbatim transcripts were made of each interview and multiple levels of interpretation were used to analyze the transcripts, first of individual interviews and then across all interviews. In addition, the participants served as the final authority, verifying or refuting the interpretation. Furthermore, comparisons were made between findings from these participants and current understandings published from other studies.

Major Concepts of Early Recognition

The first conceptual theme identified was knowing, and it was manifested as three distinct types: (1) knowing the patient, (2) knowing the patient through the family, and (3) knowing what sick looks like. "Knowing the patient" was related to how the patient typically responded and the subtle changes the nurse might notice. These findings were consistent with the findings of Benner, Tanner, and Chesla (1996). "Knowing the patient through the family" was related to slight changes the family would report to the nurse. The third theme, "knowing what sick looks like," was described by the nurses as having two possibilities. There were times when nurses indicated that something just was "not quite right." Typically, nurses would report, "something's not right" when the vital signs were very slightly changed, but the small changes in these values alone were clinically insignificant. When these data were combined with the changes in color and overall presentation of the patient, the changes took on new meaning. Usually, the nurses would recognize these subtle signs and convince others to respond. Another manifestation of "knowing what sick looks like" was identified when nurses reported knowing immediately that there was a problem and what the problem was simply by looking quickly at the patient. This immediate knowing was labeled "knowing sick."

Caring was closely related to the concept of knowing the patient. Early recognizers cared enough to notice subtle changes in patients. At times, this caring was identified by the nurse as a relationship with the patient. At other times, nurses indicated that it was more about the nurses' professional self-image. For example, nurses indicated they needed to do what a "good" nurse would do. The narratives revealed that caring, as manifested by an involved stance from the nurse, can actually heighten nurses' perceptions, thus improving assessment skills and enabling the early recognition of patient problems. This power of caring sharply contrasted with situations where the recognition of patient problems was delayed or never occurred; these situations were characterized by a detached relationship between the nurse and patient. Nurses confirmed that caring heightened their perceptions, improved assessment skills, and enabled the early recognition of patient problems (Minick, 1995).

Nurses who provided narratives of early recognition had a sense of responsibility or feelings of obligation to intervene in some way—either to collect more data or to summon the physician. Nurses never questioned whether they would respond, but only how they would respond.

The early recognizers were willing to take risks on behalf of their patients. Specifically, they had a sense of obligation to the patient that made them willing to go head to head with the physician, if necessary for the patient's welfare. They were willing to risk the potential embarrassment of being wrong and incurring anger in order to summon the help that they believed was required. In some cases, this willingness to risk self-interest was a key element in averting disaster for these patients.

Another characteristic of early recognizers was the degree of confidence they had in their assessment of the situation. Because the nurses' assessments were often not supported by technological measurements or other observers, their confidence played a critical role in successful intervention. Nurses trusted their judgment over the technology and intervened on the patient's behalf. These expert practitioners used all the data available to them, including technical data, but trusted their own judgment over technology.

Nurses considered recognition without intervention as incomplete, and therefore interventions were considered as one aspect of the concept of early recognition. Interventions manifested as: (1) further data collection and /or (2) summoning the physician. How the nurse communicated with other health providers and the willingness of the nurse to advocate for the patient were important qualitative distinctions.

PROCEDURES FOR DEVELOPMENT

Several strategies were used to develop valid items. First, the items were based on the phenomenogical studies and the theoretical matrix derived from the studies. Three nurses currently employed as medical-surgical or critical care staff nurses met over a period of about six months to discuss the concepts and develop items according to the matrix. Group process and brainstorming were used to generate and synthesize ideas. Whenever possible, the words of nurses from the preliminary data were used in the items. In order to obtain a group rather than an individual measure, the stem, "In providing care, we (most of the nurses on this unit)," was used (Verran, Gerber, & Milton, 1995; Verran, Mark, & Lamb, 1992). Knowing that some items would be discarded (Nunnally & Bernstein, 1994), three to four times the desired number of items were developed for an initial total of 53 items.

The four expert nurses and the psychometrician reviewed the items for "accuracy, appropriateness, relevance to test specifications, technical features: construction flaws, grammar, offensiveness or appearance of 'bias,' and level of readability" (Crocker & Algina, 1986, p. 71). In addition, these experts examined each item according to the relevance of the proposed theoretical structure by editing, adding, or deleting items. As a result of this review, 12 new items were added to the instrument, resulting in a total of 66 items. Based on the comments, several items were edited to increase clarity.

The variation of participants' interpretation of the terms, instructions, or questions on a survey causes random error, which has been shown to be reduced when cognitive assessment data have been used to revise instruments (DiIorio, Holcombe, Belcher, & Maibach, 1994). Therefore, cognitive assessment was used to evaluate how respondents interpreted instructions, items, and the format of the instrument. A convenience sample of 15 registered nurses (13 females and 2 males) employed in critical care (n=8) and medical surgical nursing (n=7) were asked to read each item and think aloud as they constructed the answer to the item. The individual interviews were audiotaped and transcribed verbatim. Content analysis was conducted of each transcription to "determine the person's interpretation of the question[s] and the factors related to his or her final answer" (DiIorio, et al., 1994, p. 109). Prior to field testing, the instructions, format, and items were revised as indicated by these data.

Using the 66-item survey, data gathered from a convenience sample of 451 registered nurses employed in either medical-surgical or critical care units were used to conduct an item analysis. Initially, the extent of intercorrelation among the items was determined. Items that contributed to internal consistency were retained and the remainder discarded. Items developed for the intervention component had an item-total coefficient of .25 or less, so these items were discarded. No item had an item-item coefficient of .85 or greater, indicating redundancy (Nunnally & Bernstein, 1994). Following this item analysis, an internal consistency coefficient was calculated for the remaining 48 items. Cronbach's alpha was 0.93, indicating adequate reliability. An exploratory factor analysis (PC) of 31 items revealed four factors with loadings of $\geq$ .45. Sixteen items were related to caring or commitment to the patient (factor one); six items related to knowing the patient/family (factor two); five items were related to practicing discretionary judgment; and another four items related to the notion of pattern recognition. Each of the four factors included notions of knowledge and care.

Data collection was then initiated with a second set of critical care and medical-surgical nurses ($n = 302$). Initially, the distribution and variability of each item was examined; items having little or no variability were deleted. Highly skewed items were examined for their theoretical importance and considered for deletion. The remaining 23 items were then examined for the item-to-total correlations, and those with a correlation of less than .25 or greater than .8 were deleted. The alpha coefficient for the remaining 16 items was 0.87.

The initial theoretical construct of early recognition contained four components; yet a principal component factor analysis with varimax rotation indicated a three-factor solution with loadings ranging from .572 to .827 explaining 56.9% of the variation.

DESCRIPTION

The Manifestations of Early Recognition scale (MER) is a 16-item self-report scale assessing the attributes of nurses who work together on a unit. The items measure the skill of early recognition. Although all items imply a strong commitment to care for patients/families, the items explicitly represent three dimensions, (1) knowing the patient/family, (2) knowing the system/institution and pushing the boundaries of practice to obtain what patients need, and (3) knowing the skills of self/colleagues. Respondents are asked to consider the nurses on all shifts on the unit when completing the survey, so a unit measure rather than an individual measure is reflected in the score. All items are positively worded, and respondents are asked to rate their responses on a 5–point scale, from 1 = *strongly disagree* to 5 = *strongly agree*. Eight items represent the dimension of knowing the patient/family. For example, "In providing care on this unit, we (most of the nurses on this unit) consider it important to know about patients' lives and concerns prior to hospitalization." Knowing the system or institution is reflected in four items. For example, "In providing care on this unit, we (most of the nurses on this unit) bend the rules and procedures based on the patient's/family's needs." The remaining four items represent knowing the skills of self/colleagues such as, "In providing care on this unit, we (most of the nurses on this unit) are comfortable trusting our assessments." See Appendix to this chapter for the complete scale.

ADMINISTRATION AND SCORING

The MER is a self-report measure reflecting attributes associated with the early recognition of patient problems. Two methods of administration have been used. In several studies, participants completed the survey on the unit. In a more recent study, the MER was used as a mail-out survey. In order for the MER to reflect a unit measure, (1) respondents are asked to consider all permanently assigned nurses on the unit when rating each item, (2) a response rate must be greater than 50%, and (3) an inter-unit correlation must be greater than the between-unit correlation (Verran, Gerber, & Milton, 1995; Verran, Mark, & Lamb, 1992). Responses to each item are summed to yield a total score, ranging from 16 to 80. The higher the score the higher degree of the manifestations of early recognition (MER).

RELIABILITY AND VALIDITY

Evidence for reliability and validity are presented in Table 21.1.

TABLE 21.1 Reliability and Validity Studies for the Manifestations of Early recognition Scale

Study citation	Sample and characteristics	Reliability evidence	Validity evidence
Minick, P. (1995). The power of human caring: Early recognition of patient problems. *Scholarly Inquiry for Nursing Practice: An International Journal, 9(4),* 303–321.	*Sample size:* 30 registered nurses and 40 interviews *Sample characteristics:* employed as direct care providers in critical care units; 26 Caucasians & 4 African Americans; experience in nursing 6.5–30 years with a mean of 12.8 and median of 12.5; 27 females & 3 males.	Two key participants verified the findings. Males in this study described their nursing practice differently than females.	
Minick, P. & Harvey, S. (1995). Unpublished data.	*Sample size:* 6 registered nurses *Sample characteristics:* 6 males employed in critical care as direct care providers; 5 Caucasians & one African American	Nurses in this study described their nursing practice in very similar ways to the descriptions provided by the predominantly female sample in the 1995 study.	
Minick, P. & Harvey, S. (in press). The early recognition of patient problems among medical surgical nurses *Medical-Surgical Nursing Journal.*	Sample size: 14 females; *Sample characteristics:* One African American and 13 Caucasians nurses all employed as direct care providers in medical surgical units	Medical surgical nurses described their nursing practices very similarly to those of critical care nurses.	

TABLE 21.1 *(continued)*

Study citation	Sample and characteristics	Reliability evidence	Validity evidence
Minick, P., DiIorio, C., Mitchell, P., & Dudley, W. (in development). *The early recognition of patient problems: Developing an instrument reflecting nursing expertise.*	*Sample size:* 451 registered nurses *Sample characteristics:* employed as direct care providers; 275 Caucasian, 136 African-American, 14 Asian/Pacific Ilander, 10 Other & 19 left unanswered; 415 females and 36 males		Items developed using data from qualitative studies. Content validity conducted by 4 experts.
	Sample size: 300 registered nurses *Sample characteristics:* employed as direct care providers in either critical care or medical-surgical nursing; 185 Caucasians, 74 African-Americans, 10 Asians, 3 Hispanic, 17 Other, and 5 who did not indicate; ages ranged from 22 to 60 with a mean of 37; 89.7% females, 9% male and 1.4% unanswered		In the 16 item instrument, a principle component FA revealed three constructs with factor loadings of 0.481 to 0.834 that explained 58% of the variance.

TABLE 21.1 *(continued)*

Study citation	Sample and characteristics	Reliability evidence	Validity evidence
Corley, M., Minick, P., Elswick, R. K., Jacobs, M., & McGuire, H. (2002). Nurse moral distress, nursing expertise, and ethical work environment. Submitted to Research in Nursing and Health.	*Sample size:* 160 registered nurses *Sample characteristics:* Female = 92.5% ($n = 148$); Male = 5% ($n = 8$); Not indicated = ($n = 4$); Caucasians = 112; African Americans = 30; Asian-Pacific Ilanders = 4; Other = 5; Not indicated = 9	*Internal consistency:* Cronbach's alpha = 0.88	A variance of .28 of nurses moral distress was explained by the following three interactions: (1) pushing the boundaries of practice (MER Factor 2) with experience (2) pushing the boundaries of practice with ethical environment (3) pushing the boundaries by knowing the patient (MER Factor 1)

CONCLUSIONS AND RECOMMENDATIONS

The MER was developed to measure attributes associated with the level of early recognition skills among nurses working on a particular unit. Reliability and validity assessments conducted thus far indicate that the MER meets the standards for a reliable and valid measure. Cronbach's alpha coefficients have ranged from 0.87–0.93, indicating adequate internal consistency. Factor analysis revealed three factors that did not always correspond with the preconceived structure of the instrument indicating a more complex structure than originally conceptualized.

Additional data are needed to further document the validity and reliability of the MER. Because the MER is conceptualized to reflect nursing expertise on the entire unit, then units with higher MER scores should logically have higher unit cohesion, nurse satisfaction levels and better patient outcomes when acuity is controlled. Other variables likely to influence MER scores include: (a) changes in communication patterns between nurses, (b) changes in communication patterns between nurses and physicians, and (c) changes in staffing patterns. For example, high levels of staff turnover would likely decrease the average MER score for the unit. The MER is recommended for use in clinical practice and research when a measure of expertise is needed to supplement skill-mix.

ACKNOWLEDGMENT

I would especially like to acknowledge Dr. Colleen DiIorio's guidance in developing this instrument.

REFERENCES

Benner, P., Hooper-Kyriakidis, P., & Stannard, D. S. (1999). *Clinical wisdom and interventions in critical-care: A thinking-in-action approach.* Philadelphia: W. B. Saunders.

Benner, P., Tanner, C., & Chesla, C. (1996). *Expertise in nursing practice: Caring, clinical judgment, and ethics.* New York: Springer Publishing Co.

Benner, P., & Wrubel, J. (1989). *The primacy of caring: Stress and coping in health and illness.* Menlo Park, CA: Addison-Wesley. Corley, M., Minick, P., Elswick, R. K., Jacobs, M., & McGuire, H. (2002). Nurse moral distress, nursing expertise, and ethical work environment. Submitted to *Research in Nursing and Health.*

Crocker, L., & Algina, J. (1986). *Introduction to classical & modern test theory.* Philadelphia: Harcourt Brace Jovanovich College Publishers.

DiIorio, C., Holcombe, J., Belcher, L., & Maibach, E. (1994). Use of cognitive assessment method to evaluate the adequacy of sexually transmitted disease history questions. *Journal of Nursing Measurement, 2*(2), 107–116.

Hamers, J., Huijer Abu Saad, H., & Halfens, R. (1994). Diagnostic process and decision making in nursing: Literature review. *Journal of Professional Nursing, 10*(3), 154–163.

Jenny, J., & Logan, J. (1992). Knowing the patient: One aspect of clinical knowledge. *Image: Journal of Nursing Scholarship, 24,* 254–258.

Minick, P. (1995). The power of human caring: The early recognition of patient problems. *Scholarly Inquiry for Nursing Practice, 9,* 303–321.

Minick, P., DiIorio, C., Mitchell, P., & Dudley, W. (2002) The early recognition of patient problems: Development an instrument reflecting nursing expertise.

Minick, P., & Harvey, S. (in press). The early recognition of patient problems among medical–surgical nurses. *Medical Surgical Nursing Journal.*

Nunnally, J., & Bernstein, I. (1994). *Psychometric theory,* 3rd Edition. New York: McGraw-Hill.

Verran, J., Gerber, R., & Milton, D. (1995). Data aggregation: Criteria for psychometric evaluation. *Research in Nursing and Health, 18*(1), 77–80.

Verran, J., Mark, B., & Lamb, G. (1992). Psychometric examination of instruments using aggregated data. *Research in Nursing and Health, 15,* 237–240.

APPENDIX: MANIFESTATIONS OF EARLY RECOGNITION OF PATIENT PROBLEMS

Instructions: Please indicate how you and most of your colleagues on this unit would typically respond while providing direct patient care.

In providing care, we (most of the nurses on this unit):	Strongly Disagree	Somewhat Disagree	Somewhat Agree	Agree	Strongly Agree
1. are able to act on our own judgments without input from another nurse or physician most of the time.	1	2	3	4	5
2. are comfortable trusting our assessments when technology suggests the contrary.	1	2	3	4	5
3. do something other than what standard practice is if we feel a patient needs it.	1	2	3	4	5
4. feel that knowing the personal aspects of a patient is important.	1	2	3	4	5
5. try to understand how the patient views his/her illness.	1	2	3	4	5
6. consider it important to know "who" the patients are as people.	1	2	3	4	5
7. are able to recognize very subtle changes in patient status us.	1	2	3	4	5
8. try to understand how the patient and family interacted prior to the hospitalization.	1	2	3	4	5
9. consider it important to know about patients' lives and their concerns prior to admission.	1	2	3	4	5
10. bend the rules and procedures based on the patients' needs.	1	2	3	4	5
11. will continue to seek clarification/question the physician when an order does not quite make sense.	1	2	3	4	5
12. become involved with patient/families to provide better care.	1	2	3	4	5
13. try to determine the wishes of patient/families.	1	2	3	4	5
14. know from experience what is important to observe or notice in the patient.	1	2	3	4	5
15. now what to expect, because we frequently care for the same kinds of patient/family problems.	1	2	3	4	5
16. frequently push the boundaries of nursing to obtain whatever the patient and family need.	1	2	3	4	5

Index

Weisman, A.D., 97
Weiss, C., 157, 235, 236, 240
    S.J., 161
Welch-McCaffrey, D., 212, 213
Wells, D., 57, 61
Wells, N., 187, 194
Wheeler, K., 207, 208, 209, 210, 211, 213

Whitmer, K., 116
Witkin, H.A., 196
Witter, J., 225
Wood, R., 48

Yeagley, S.C., 80, 81